From his pastor's heart, Jim Henry  vith biblical passages from God's Word ; of all those who travel alongside their the journey of Alzheimer's disease, and oi .... ucpenuency upon the God of all comfort.

—FRANKLIN GRAHAM
PRESIDENT & CEO, BILLY GRAHAM EVANGELISTIC ASSOCIATION
AND SAMARITAN'S PURSE

With his pastoral heart, Jim Henry addresses one of the real-life challenges that families face as they are confronted with becoming caregivers for their loved ones. This book is practical and helpful, but also overflowing with hope. I recommend this book to all persons, all churches, all businesses, and all organizations who have a heart to help others who are caring for their loved ones.

—DR. RONNIE FLOYD
PRESIDENT & CEO, SOUTHERN BAPTIST CONVENTION EXECUTIVE
COMMITTEE

Using practical, common-sense counsel gleaned from his walk with his wife who suffered with Alzheimer's, Dr. Jim Henry helps us to understand what is happening in this dark journey in which the patient never gets better and the caregivers never get rest, and to make the long journey more compassionate and comfortable. My family, too, has been touched by this scourge.

—GOVERNOR MIKE HUCKABEE, AR 1996–2007
HOST OF "HUCKABEE" ON TBN; FOX NEWS CONTRIBUTOR

A *must-read* for any family caring for a loved one suffering from Alzheimer's or dementia, and the challenges associated with the disease. Rev. Jim Henry, caregiver for his wife, Jeanette, and Deb Terry who cared for her father, Ray, take readers behind the scenes, offering great advice on how to confront the most difficult aspects of this very prevalent disease.

—Bob Clement, former U.S. Congressman–TN
Life-long friend of Jim and Jeanette

Deb Terry and Dr. Jim Henry take us on a deeply, personal and heart-wrenching, yet hopeful, story of their experiences with Alzheimer's disease. This book is biblically based, practical, raw, and down to earth. In my opinion, it is for families on this journey (or have gone through it), and for all others impacted by Alzheimer's. I especially recommend it to pastors.

—H. Wilson Nelson, D. Min.
Retired Pastor, University Administrator and Coach

As the dreaded diagnosis of Alzheimer's spreads to more of our loved ones, Pastor Jim Henry's message could not be more timely. Borne of his personal experience and lifelong faith, his words provide needed understanding, comfort, and direction for all who are touched by this tragic illness.

—Bill Frederick
Mayor Emeritus of Orlando

Many resources offer facts and information, but this book, in addition to offering advice, speaks to the heart and blesses the soul. My friend and partner in ministry, Deb Terry, has poured her faith and experience into this book because she wants to help you in coping with the unimaginable.

—Tim Grosshans
Pastor, First Baptist Church of Winter Garden, Florida

JIM HENRY
DEB TERRY

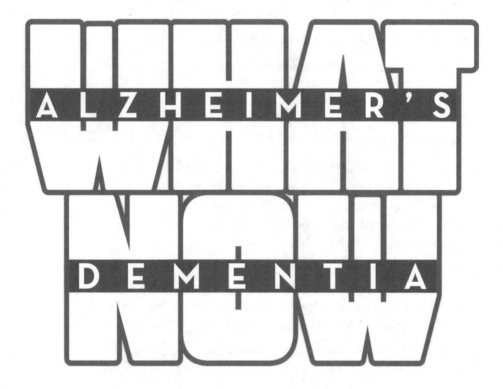

WHAT
ALZHEIMER'S
NOW
DEMENTIA

HELP AND HOPE FOR
CAREGIVERS, FAMILY, AND FRIENDS

Alzheimer's, Dementia. What Now?
Help and Hope for Caregivers, Family, and Friends

© 2020 Jim Henry and Deb Terry. All rights reserved.

ISBN-13: 978-1-951492-86-1 paperback
ISBN: 978-1-951492-17-5 eBook
Library of Congress case no. 1-8588790011

Published by: HigherLife Development Services, Inc.
PO Box 623307
Oviedo, FL 32762
(407) 563-4806
www.ahigherlife.com

No part of this book may be reproduced without written permission from the publisher or copyright holder, nor may any part of this book be transmitted in any form or by any means electronic, mechanical, photocopying, recording, or other, without prior written permission from the publisher or copyright holder.

Unless otherwise noted, Scripture quotations are from the Holy Bible, New International Version, copyright © 2011 by Zondervan Publishing Company. NIV® Copyright © 1973, 1978, 1984, 2011, 2019 by Biblica, Inc.® Used by permission. All rights reserved worldwide.

The Message Bible MSG. ©1993–2002 permission of the publisher, NavPress Publishing Group.

The Holy Bible, English Standard Version. ESV® Text Edition: 2016. Copyright © 2001 by Crossway Bibles, a publishing ministry of Good News Publishers.

Cover Design: Dee DeLoy

Printed in the United States of America
10 9 8 7 6 5 4 3 2 1

TABLE OF CONTENTS

SECTION I:
WHEN THE DIAGNOSIS IS MADE

SECTION II:
WHEN THE DISEASE TAKES OVER

PREFACE

Jim Henry's Experience Having a Spouse with Alzheimer's Disease

While sitting in a nice restaurant in Orlando with my wife, Jeanette, I noticed a couple who was seated diagonally across from us. When their food came, the man began to feed the woman in much the same manner a parent would feed a small child. Fork by fork, followed by sips of water, he patiently fed her and occasionally spoke to her. I wondered why he was feeding her, as it seemed she had no physical problems. I watched her as she ate. She was mechanically chewing, not speaking, showing no facial expressions, and staring blankly.

Later I became all too familiar with this kind of scenario and that blank stare. It was the look of dementia. The feeding routine I saw would be mine one day with my beautiful Jeanette.

Strangely, it was around food when we began to notice Jeanette's early stage Alzheimer's. At restaurants she had difficulty in choosing her food. This was unusual for her as she was always decisive in all areas of life. The wonderful asset of decision-making is one of chief robbers of reality in Alzheimer's world.

That world quietly invaded ours in December 2012 at the office of our internist, where we had gone for our yearly check-up. Because he suspected some change in Jeanette's cognitive function and factored in a family history of some memory loss issues on Jeanette's father's side of the family, our internist suggested we might go to a couple of doctors for some tests. He also made a follow-up appointment for us to see him again for some memory tests.

Two weeks later I got a call from Jeanette while I was driving to Tallahassee for a Sunday preaching engagement. She was having a panic attack. Our daughter Betsy dashed over to the house to be with her. She reported that her mom was having a tough time concentrating and remembering things.

On New Year's Eve 2012 I wrote in my journal:

> *Now a New Year—what lies before us? All is in my Father's hands.*

Things seemed to be normal with Jeanette for a few weeks until one January evening in 2013 when she could not recall having eaten ice cream twice that day. She thought she had eaten it the prior night. As we talked, it was evident that she had no recollection of many past events.

Later that night I wrote in my journal:

> *"The Lord replied, 'My Presence will go with you, and I will give you rest'" (Exodus 33:14).*

I was to lean on His Presence many times in the days ahead.

In February, we celebrated Valentine's Day at one of our favorite restaurants where Jeanette gave me a card on which these words were penned, "The only one I will ever love." Similar words she wrote me four years later even though she was entering the early part of her last stage of Alzheimer's.

In March Jeanette mentioned she was worried about not being able to remember names. She said she had seen "ten or twelve people at church and could not recall a single name." Jeanette went on to express concern over her memory lapses. For the first time she mentioned the word *dementia.* I tried to steer the conversation by saying maybe some of her medications were affecting her recall.

That evening I wrote in my journal:

> *Lord, if she is going that way, let me live to take care of her.*

Later that month our daughter Betsy called and said, "Dad, we need to talk. I, other family members, and close friends have observed..." what

Jeanette and I had discussed. Her timing was interesting as I was just getting ready to text her when she called me.

Betsy and I met and compared notes. The next day Betsy came over to the house so we could share our mutual concerns with Jeanette, which is what Jeanette's doctor had encouraged us to do. Jeanette took it stoically.

Betsy did some research on the internet and found out a thyroid problem or some medications could cause dementia-like symptoms. I embraced these possibilities and fervently prayed, *"Lord, let it be something else."* I grappled with my thoughts and emotions. I could hardly imagine losing her to this insidious disease.

Some days later Jeanette was lying on the couch and asked me twice what I was doing tomorrow. Then she blurted out, "Jim, if I have dementia, our lives will be changed."

"If you do, I will be here for you," I assured her.

What Jeanette said became our reality. Our lives were dramatically changed in the coming days and years.

About a week later, Jeanette went to her appointment with her psychiatrist. Afterwards I asked, "How did it go?"

"Not a good report," she said. "I did not do well on the memory part. He is sending me to a neurologist and for an MRI." She began to cry.

I held her close and prayed as the cold reality of the journey we were about to share soaked in. I then went to the only place I knew to go, that is, to my heavenly Father on my knees. There I prayed: *Father, help my Jeanette glorify your Name. Grant me courage, faith, strength, no self-pity, and to be there for her. If this is the beginning of the long journey into twilight, dusk, and heaven, I trust You. My eyes look to You, Our Presence.*

By April the memory lapses were increasingly worse. The visit with the neurologist found her unable to remember three words he asked her to recall or draw a clock to show the time of 11:10. When we got in our car after the appointment, Jeanette was full of questions and could not remember the doctor's name.

Days later, another neurologist gave her a test that lasted three-and-a-half hours. He told me he could prescribe some meds that

DEB TERRY'S EXPERIENCE HAVING A PARENT WITH ALZHEIMER'S DISEASE

I will never forget the call I received November 16, 2006. I was sitting in my office when my mom, June, called to tell me the results of my dad's visit to the doctor. "The doctor said he has Alzheimer's."

My whole body felt the weight of that statement. I could only respond, "I'm so sorry and I love you."

After talking with my mom, my upper body folded on my desk and I begin to weep. My dad, Ray, was seventy-four years old when he was diagnosed with advanced Alzheimer's. I knew very little about the disease. However, I knew enough to know this is not good and there is no cure.

After my tears, I gathered my thoughts and felt a passion rise from within me to learn all I could about this horrible disease. I vowed to do everything I possibly could: read, research, and talk with people who knew more than I did about this disease, so that I could help my family care for my dad.

I knew working a full-time job and living almost six-hundred miles from my parents and brother would present a challenge. As my husband and I processed this life-altering diagnosis, we prayed that God would give us wisdom on how to best help my family. For months we earnestly sought answers to our constant prayers.

Finally, God clearly spoke to our hearts with the direction we should take. I resigned from my position as the children's director at First Baptist Church of Orlando. My husband, Scott, also made a career decision that facilitated our moving to take care of my dad. My husband's boss created a new territory in Alabama that allowed Scott to keep his job. An action plan was in place. Our house sold in two weeks. We moved April 8, 2007.

Scott and I entered a world about which we knew very little and started a journey only God could help us navigate. We began with no specific plan in mind of how to care for Dad. However, we were certain God had a plan. God faithfully revealed what we needed day by day and step by step as we put our trust in Him to take care of our needs.

My brother, Steve, was instrumental in taking precautions to protect my parents' assets and make sound financial decisions while my dad was able. Because my brother and Dad had been in business together, it became much easier for financial decisions to be made. This brought great peace of mind to my mother. The last thing she needed to be thinking about was finances. However, financial planning is critical in taking care of a loved one with Alzheimer's. Our family found being proactive and staying ahead of the disease helped make decisions less stressful and more manageable.

I often wondered if my dad's life experiences came into play with this disease. Born in 1932 as the youngest of three children, my dad stepped up early to care for his disabled mother after his parents' divorce. His heart was always set on providing help and protection for his mother. I believe he saw things kids should never see as there was constant fear in his home. While Dad was an eager learner and hard worker, he was only able to complete the eighth grade as he needed to work a full-time job to support the two of them. Not only did his mother need him, eventually, his country did, as well.

At age 17, he joined the National Guard and was deployed at age 19 to serve on the front lines in the Korean War. His best friend, who was fighting beside him, was killed in a horrific way, which was etched in his mind forever. He constantly struggled to suppress the emotions triggered by those memories. This traumatic experience changed him as a young man, as did other horrendous experiences he never shared with anyone, except once or twice with my mom. Because he never wanted to talk about those experiences again, he did not register with the Veteran's Administration to be in their system. This decision later prevented him from receiving care in a V.A. hospital during his battle with Alzheimer's.

Upon returning from the war, my dad, Ray, started his own business: a wholesale car dealership. He was in his twenties when he started it up. Dad was good with his hands, had a strong work ethic, and possessed keen business savvy, all of which contributed to his becoming a very successful businessman. He met June, a beautiful young woman, introduced by one of her relatives and a friend of my dad's. They married six weeks after meeting and began their family—having two children, including my brother and me. My dad's car business provided a great living for our family and helped prepare him for early retirement, and eventually funded his care and my mom's future. Over the years Dad played many sports and games, some competitively, including table tennis and checkers. He also loved music, especially playing the guitar, which he played quite well.

A few years after my dad's retirement, we started noticing some things were different with him. He began to show signs of memory issues. He struggled with balancing the checkbook, getting lost, and becoming easily agitated when unable to perform tasks he was accustomed to doing. Loss of confidence and fear began to overtake his thinking. Dad no longer wanted to do anything or go anywhere that was unfamiliar. He backed away from participating in activities, conversations, travel, and many other things he loved. Even though he had not yet been diagnosed with Alzheimer's, we could not help but notice his memory issues were progressing.

Due to Dad's strong physical physique as a six-foot, 175-pound, seventy-four-year-old man, we knew he may be difficult to handle. Yet, as a family, we were committed to care for him at home as long as we could. It was a challenge—a challenge that became increasingly more difficult over time. My dad could never settle down or be content. He constantly wanted to "get out" of wherever he was and go home. He rarely sat down or rested. Dad always wanted to walk, stay on the go, and do things he should not.

When the difficult got even more difficult, we knew taking care of my father was more than we could handle on our own. Our family had done the best we could do with the resources, extended family, friends, and medical help. However, we had reached the point where we were beginning to exhaust all our local options.

Would we have done anything differently? I do not know. I do know we gave our best. Each month we faced new challenges that caused us to recalibrate and prepare as best we could for whatever was next. However, with this disease it is impossible to predict what will come next.

Our family quickly learned how exhausting it is to be caregivers. We discovered there are people, organizations, facilities, and professional caregivers available. Once we sought their assistance, we were blessed with wonderful caregivers including primary care physicians, hospice professionals, nurses, social workers, sitters, as well as the medical directors and staffs of facilities where my dad lived for almost two years.

It has now been a decade since my dad passed. He no longer battles this horrible disease that took him from being a handsome, smart, loving man to becoming a shadow of his former self whom we hardly recognized as our beloved Ray. Over the years, I have had many opportunities to tell our story and help others along the way. I have often been asked, "Do you have a book, or do you plan to write one?"

God's perfect provision and timing allowed Dr. Jim Henry and me to collaborate on this project. We found much commonality in our experiences of walking with a loved one through the ravages of this horrible disease. There are lessons we both have learned through this process that will help others gain insight, offer hope in times of despair, and point to the kind of healing only God can provide.

Our message to you, the caregiver, is to take heart. You are not alone!

INTRODUCTION

WHY WE WROTE THIS BOOK

Y OU'RE IN FOR a wild ride!" Our physician remarked when Jeanette, my wife of fifty-four years, and I were getting the results of our yearly checkups. He went on to tell me things I should observe about Jeanette. He then said, "If it's dementia, it will be like riding a rollercoaster."

His words hung in the air as if attached to an invisible rope. I was stunned! I did not know how to begin to respond. In that devastating moment, the only thing I could think to do was pray. We prayed right there before leaving his office.

Most of my life, I have been a caregiver for God's people. Now I was being called to be a caregiver for the one person to whom I was most important—the love of my life, who has stood by me and with me. She loved me unconditionally as my helper and the caregiver for our family. I was entering a world about which I knew very little. I did not have a clue about what I needed to do or what I needed to know to assume this role.

However, I do know this now. That is why this book was written. Our journey took off on that wild rollercoaster ride. Yours may have just begun or, perhaps, you have been on this ride for a while. This book is intended to encourage you on your journey as you care for your loved one while walking each step of "the long good-bye."

While my co-author, Deb Terry, and I have experienced caring for a loved one with Alzheimer's, we are not medical professionals. While we have done research in seeking ways to better look after our loved ones, we do not profess to be experts in the care and treatment of this awful disease. Our hope is to share practical advice and personal experiences in the hope we can help lighten your load as you are trying to make sense of what you are facing.

Assuming the role of caregiver of a loved one with AD is more than a wild ride. Your ride will have innumerable ups and downs, twists and turns, fear inducing moments, and times when your heart sinks. You may feel overwhelmed or want to get off the ride. However, without trivializing what you are experiencing, we want to encourage you to hold on and finish the ride. Our experience has taught us this ride has the potential to change your life in positive and healing ways.

There is hope, so please do not despair. Let us help you through this. The same heavenly Father to whom I turned in my time of need is there to offer you help and hope to see it through to the end. You can count on it.

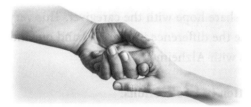

Scripture: "As my heart grows faint; lead me to the Rock that is higher than I" (Psalm 61:2).

Prayer: *Father, I feel overwhelmed by what lies before me. You are my Rock. You will lead me. You are enough. Thank you.*

How This Book Is Organized

This is written for individuals who have a loved one with AD, which is an abbreviation we are going to use in this book to designate Alzheimer's disease and other types of advanced dementia with symptoms similar to Alzheimer's. We pray this book will help you in your role as caregiver for your loved one. This book revolves around *18 Central Questions* for which you are (or will be) seeking answers and guidance while on this journey.

STAGE ONE SYMPTOMS OF ALZHEIMER'S DISEASE:

MILD OR EARLY STAGE

- Exhibiting short-term memory loss
- Becoming forgetful with names and places
- Forgetting how to use numbers (e.g., phone, television remote, check writing, credit cards)
- Daily tasks and organization becoming more challenging
- Reading problems
- Declining object recognition
- Increasingly poor sense of direction

QUESTION #1:

WHAT ARE THE FIRST THINGS I NEED TO KNOW?

THERE ARE NATURAL changes that occur in the body, including the brain, during the aging process. With age, people may not be as physically strong or mentally sharp as in previous years. Someone may display signs of mild forgetfulness, such as having trouble remembering someone's name. However, if given some time or prompting, the name comes to mind, which is completely normal.

If your loved one's memory problems are more dramatically impacting his or her daily life, then it behooves you both to consider the possibility that he or she may be showing the early signs of AD (Alzheimer's disease or another type of dementia). Although this is an unbelievably scary prospect, it is far better to face this possibility head on rather than letting fear keep you from moving forward. The sooner you get a medical diagnosis, the sooner your loved one may start treatment to help relieve symptoms and allow you time to prepare for the future.

ACKNOWLEDGING YOUR LOVED ONE MAY HAVE AD

Take note of these early signs of Alzheimer's, some of which may be symptoms of other types of dementia:[1]

1. *Displaying Progressive Memory Loss*

You may have noticed your loved one's memory progressively failing over an extended period of time. Is your loved one forgetting the names of close friends or family? Is your loved one increasingly forgetting important dates? Are they forgetting information he or she just learned? Have you observed the pattern of his or her habitually asking for the same information over and over?

2. *Showing Difficulty with Problem Solving*

Early signs may include your noticing your loved one can no longer do something they formerly have been able to do. For example, they may be having trouble following directions, as in preparing a recipe; keeping track of personal finances, as in balancing a checking account; making decisions, as when ordering from a restaurant menu; or using electronic devices, as when using the phone or television remote.

3. *Demonstrating Challenges with Routine Tasks*

Is your loved one having trouble driving to a familiar location? Do they get disoriented or lost easily, such as in a store or at the mall? Are they forgetting the rules of a favorite sport or how to play a favorite game? Are they losing things or putting household items in places that make no sense? For example, Jeanette put my socks in the dishwasher.

4. *Struggling with Verbal Communication*

Beyond forgetting important names, dates, or information recently acquired, is your loved one having an increasingly difficult time expressing their thoughts? Are they calling things by the wrong name? For example, Jeanette would call the street the "trail." The post office became the "letter house."

5. *Revealing Lapses in Judgment*

Is your loved one making poor decisions? Are they still handling their money and possessions with appropriate wisdom? Are they taking inappropriate risks with their safety and physical well-being? Are they making healthy food and substance choices? Are their personal hygiene practices declining? Are they dressing for appropriate weather or occasions?

6. *Exhibiting Patterns of Social Withdrawal*

Has your loved one begun to withdraw from former enjoyable activities or hobbies? Does your loved one prefer staying home and watching television or sleeping instead of going out of the house to be around others or do something stimulating?

7. *Displaying Mood Changes*

Does your loved one show uncharacteristic signs of depression or anxiety? Are they getting upset more quickly and often? Have they become irrationally afraid of being wronged or harmed?

8. *Evidencing Trouble with Vision*

Are you noticing a decline in your loved one's vision? Are they still judging distances as well as they formerly did? Are they bumping into things more often? Are they walking differently?

Deb's Experience:

Although my dad was seventy-four years old when he was diagnosed with Alzheimer's, he probably could have been diagnosed in his late sixties. Because he retired when he was sixty-three years old and no longer in a work setting, it was more difficult to recognize all the little things with which he was having difficulty. My mom knew something was not quite right with my dad's memory. However, she did not know it was Alzheimer's. She often would cover for him to keep him from being embarrassed when he would forget a name, what to say, or what to do. My mom began noticing he was no longer confident in making decisions. She began to question his judgement in driving. Also, he no longer wanted to travel or be away from home, which was something he enjoyed doing for many years.

During one of the last trips they took with friends to a very familiar area, he got lost looking for their hotel room. He did not know how to use the elevator or remember what floor they were staying on. His friends noticed he had a hard time deciding and ordering his meal.

My parents both knew he was changing. However, they did not know exactly what was happening. My dad, who had been an astute businessman, could no longer balance a checkbook. He began to misplace things. He would start looking for something and then forget what he was searching for. Then, if he found the object, he could not remember how to use it. This was becoming his new normal. My mom knew it was time to see their family doctor, who was also a close friend, who could help them begin to navigate their journey with Alzheimer's.

While your loved one may not have all these early signs of AD or all to the same degree, it is important that you take note of these changes and the frequency of their occurrence. If you find yourself in the position where your loved one's uncharacteristic behavior or memory lapses are occurring more frequently, make an appointment with their primary care physician.

Preparing for and Sharing Your Concerns with the Doctor

Here are some helpful tips when preparing to speak with your loved one's doctor:

- Prior to visiting the doctor, contact your loved one's doctor with your concerns.

- It is important you protect your loved one's feelings regarding an Alzheimer's suspicion or diagnosis. While the prospect of confirming your worst suspicions will be extremely difficult for you, it will be devastating for your loved one.

- Accompany your loved one to see their doctor.

- It is important for you to go with your loved one to see their doctor to help present a more complete picture of what has changed and what symptoms are occurring more frequently.

- Share your observations, as well as a time line of the frequency of symptoms displayed.

- Help provide a complete medical history.

- Help the doctor to identify any other possible illnesses or medical problems (e.g., stroke) that may be mimicking AD symptoms or causing your loved one's AD to progress more rapidly and need to be addressed and treated.

- Request early testing instead of waiting.

In addition to a physical exam, the doctor should perform tests of their mental status: memory, verbal skills, problem solving, thinking skills, and mood. Early testing takes the guess work out of the equation. Ask for the F.A.S.T. Test (Functional Assessment Staging Test). This test determines at what stage of the disease one is. Early diagnosis can help in making the best plan to provide the best care for your loved one. Recognizing and accepting this early on will be helpful in each stage.

- Your doctor may order additional tests.

- Your doctor may order imaging tests of the brain—an MRI or PET scan—to help make a diagnosis of Alzheimer's. These are expensive tests. Medicare and some other insurance providers may not cover these diagnostic tests.

FINDING AND ENLISTING THE HELP OF MEDICAL SPECIALISTS

Your doctor may refer your loved one to a medical professional who specializes in dementia to test your loved one and get an accurate diagnosis.[2] If your loved one is sixty-five years of age or older, it will be helpful to have them tested and evaluated by a neurologist specializing in geriatrics.

Family members often try to diagnose their loved one with Alzheimer's disease when it may not be this at all. A memory issue can be one of many types of dementia. Getting the correct medical diagnosis is most important in the care of your loved one.

- One dementia support group estimates there are over 400 different types of dementia;[3] however, most sources identify and focus on fewer than five, ten, or twenty common types of dementia.

- Dementia is a *syndrome* (i.e., a group of symptoms which do not lead to a specific diagnosis).

- Dementia is used as an umbrella term to describe symptoms that impact memory and functioning.[4]

- Alzheimer's disease is a type of dementia. It is the most common type of dementia, affecting one in ten Americans over the age of 65.[5]

It can be difficult to determine what type of dementia your loved one may be experiencing. The only way to accurately secure a diagnosis is to see the medical specialist(s) and have medical tests performed as your doctor(s) may advise. Do not hesitate to ask questions of your doctor or specialist who will help you learn about this disease. Throughout the diagnostic process continue to keep your health providers informed of changes in your loved one's health, memory, and functioning.

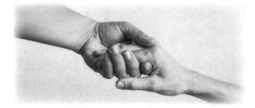

Scripture: "For you do not know what a day will bring forth" (Proverbs 27:1).

Prayer: *God, we did not expect this day, but it has come. We are struggling to come to grips with it. Help us.*

QUESTION #2:

WHAT ARE THE FIRST STEPS I NEED TO TAKE?

Processing the diagnosis of Alzheimer's will take time and soul searching. The process of acceptance is just as important for you as it is your loved one. It is hard and heart-breaking for both of you. As there will be no perfect ending, there are no perfect steps to take in commencing this new life journey.

Allow Yourself Time to Grieve

- You and your loved one may need time to grieve over the loss of the future you have envisioned.

- It is normal to feel great sadness when facing this horrible disease.

- Fear and feeling alone in handling this without your loved one's help are common emotions you will experience.

Accept the Diagnosis

- You will not want to believe the diagnosis.

- Denial will not be helpful in caring for your loved one.

- You may need time to process the new diagnosis and begin envisioning yourself as a caregiver. However, you must move forward with this journey one step at a time.

Learn All You Can About the Disease

- Be resourceful in researching and gathering as much information about Alzheimer's as you can.

- The more you read and learn, the better equipped you will be in understanding how best to help your loved one and yourself.

- Some have called Alzheimer's "the longest funeral." The average life expectancy after diagnosis is eight to ten years. However, Alzheimer's can last as long as twenty years.[1]

> **Deb's Experience:**
>
> *One day while we were still caring for my dad at their home, I took him to a nearby state park, which was a favorite place of his. While I drove the back roads, my dad gave me precise directions and never missed a turn. However, two hours later when we sat down to play a game of checkers—a game that he had played competitively in previous years—he could not remember how to play.*

It is heart-breaking to watch someone lose their mental capacity as you will be affected by the dramatic changes that occur as you watch your loved one struggle with daily tasks and their altered interactions with others. Alzheimer's disease starts with mild memory loss and ends with total memory loss.

Understanding and caring for your loved one may be extraordinarily difficult. You must learn to communicate with them in a different way. As the disease progresses, you may need to learn to be your loved one's translator as they struggle to express their thoughts and feelings in the correct way. For example, Jeanette would rub her arms and say, "My windows are cold." We had to learn to begin listening for what she meant to say rather than just hearing the words that came out of her mouth.

In the later stage of her disease, Jeanette asked our daughter Betsy why she was "in jail." Jeanette did not know what she did wrong. Greatly saddened by Jeanette's perception of her situation and her inability to communicate well with us, we surmised that Jeanette was trying to express the way she was feeling—trapped—and not being able to properly voice how she felt.

It is good to talk with others who are dealing with or who have dealt with caring for a loved one with Alzheimer's. Do not be embarrassed to share your experience with this disease or ask questions. When talking about a loved one who is dealing with memory issues, it is helpful to know (and remember) that Alzheimer's is not a mental issue, rather a disease of the brain that affects the memory.

Deb's Experience:

Because of my personality, gifts, and passion, I found myself doing a lot of research—mainly utilizing the research and resources provided by the Alzheimer's Association—to make sure I had up-to-date and accurate information on this disease so that I could share the information with my family. If I found a highly recommended book, I would order three: one for my mom, my brother, and me. This was helpful for all of us to be reading and learning together to help care for the man we all loved so deeply.

Keep a Journal

- It is important that you keep a journal, writing down notes and dates of the things you notice that are different with your loved one. This will allow you to track their frequency.

- Journaling will be more helpful than you can imagine as your loved one's disease progresses. Not only will it be extremely useful for medical purposes, but it will be therapeutic for you as the caregiver.

- You may think you will remember all the details, but that is not the case as this journey is long and taxing.

Plus, your emotional and physical state will compound difficulty in remembering everything you will want or need to recall.

My practice of journaling helped me throughout Jeanette's illness, especially as I tried to process what was happening and its impact on both of us.

On May 17, 2017, I journaled:

> *Really shadowing me. Doesn't want me out of sight. Thinks we have a room "upstairs," which we do not. Having more trouble making sense with sentences and grasping for the right words to describe objects. Just heart-rending, and I cannot overcome it. Wonder if I should pray for the Lord to reverse it—has it ever happened?*

Discuss and Work Out a Treatment Plan with Doctor(s)

- If medications are prescribed for your loved one, ask questions about the efficacy, side-effects, and expense of these medications.

- Accurately share information about other medications your loved may be taking with the doctor(s) in consideration of drug interactions.

- Some medications are very expensive and may be cost prohibitive. If this is the case, ask your physician about an alternate treatment plan.

- Keep records of how your loved one responds to these meds. Are they helping your loved one or not?

- Not all medication may be helpful for your loved one.

- Some medications can complicate things and make conditions worsen.

- Do not hesitate to contact your loved one's physician(s), share your observations, and speak up if you feel the medications need to be changed or discontinued.

Jeanette met with a neurologist in April of 2013. After some brief tests, he ordered bloodwork. On May 6 we returned for our follow-up appointment. The neurologist told us Jeanette had the pathology of Alzheimer's disease. He prescribed two medications: Namenda® and the Exelon® patch to treat the cognitive symptoms of the disease—memory loss, confusion, and problems with thinking and reasoning.

Jeanette immediately began taking these prescribed medications. However, they offered her little relief. In fact, she got worse having panic attacks, getting little sleep, and feeling very insecure.

A few weeks later we took her to her psychiatrist, who had treated her for years for panic attacks. He prescribed some new meds and changed the dosage on others. This seemed to alleviate her panic attacks. Xanax®, buspirone, and risperidone were some of the prescription medications.

During the course of her illness we returned for a couple of visits to tweak dosages. He was most helpful and did more than our neurologist to assist her with her mental anguish, which may not be the case for your loved one.

Early on, the possibility of an MRI was suggested to plot what was happening in Jeanette's brain. However, the six-thousand-dollar, out-of-pocket charge for this test was too hefty for us as it could do nothing to improve her mental deficiencies.

While there is no known cure for Alzheimer's, your loved one may need medications in the beginning stage for slowing the progression of the disease and throughout the course of the disease to help relieve some of its symptoms. Your doctor can discuss specific drugs and treatment plans to help your loved one.

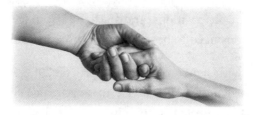

Scripture: "I will instruct you and teach you in the way you should go" (Psalm 32:8).

Prayer: *Father, so many questions, so few answers. I stand on Your promise to teach me the way to go. Thank You.*

QUESTION #3:

HOW DO I SHARE
THE DIAGNOSIS?

G ETTING THE PHYSICIAN'S diagnosis that your loved one does, indeed, have Alzheimer's disease is difficult to process. Discussing that life-changing diagnosis with your loved one is beyond difficult. Sharing that devastating diagnosis with others makes it all too real and permanent.

DISCUSSING THE DIAGNOSIS
WITH MY LOVED ONE, THE PATIENT

I really struggled with discussing Jeanette's diagnosis with her. Should I tell her in her coherent moments, which would make dealing it terribly agonizing for her? Or should I not tell her and let the ravages of the disease gradually take its toll so she might be spared from knowing what was happening?

As it turned out, she began to suspect something was changing in her life. In the summer of 2013 it began to unravel, which I documented in my journal:

June 13: After our visits to two neurologists, she asked "Do I have dementia?" for the first time.

June 29: She asked, "Am I going crazy? Do I have dementia?"

July 9: The questions continued: "Are you holding anything back from me? Will I get better?"

July 18: "I am not getting better. You've got to do something," she pled.

July 24: Trying to explain what she was experiencing, she said, "I feel drugged. I do not understand what's happening."

August 2: Trying to grab on to some hope, she asked, "Will the new pills restore my short-term memory?"

August 6: She read the Namenda prescription info that said it was for Alzheimer's and asked, "Do I have Alzheimer's?"

August 15: She came out on our porch and said, "Jim, I am losing my memory, aren't I?" She then sat in the chair and cried. I held her and told her we would fight it together.

August 18: She finally asked, "How many family and friends know I have dementia?" Then she added, "I do not want things to end this way. I love you so much."

August 22: She called me into the bedroom and said, "I've got something to talk to you about. I'm losing my mind. I've got to teach you how to pay bills and handle business."

I would also note that about this time she began to hide her wedding rings and some of her jewelry out of the fear someone was going to break into our house and steal them. Over the next months she increasingly wanted to stay at home, where she could see me, be with me, sit close to me, and clutch my hand.

I encourage you to take the opportunity to have conversations with your loved one about their changing world and significant matters while they are still able to process what is happening and are capable of communicating with you. You both may only have a narrow window of time to express your mutual support for each other, say things that need to be said, and discuss important life choices. There will be no better time to reassure your loved one they are not alone in facing their diagnosis.

> **Deb's Experience:**
>
> *When my dad's geriatric neurologist told him he could no longer drive, it was hard for my dad. It was a sad day when he cleaned out his truck with my brother and handed Steve the keys. My dad had to learn how to depend on others—my mom, family members, and friends—to drive him places. This was especially difficult for him as he loved his independence.*

It is important to allow your loved one to grieve over the impending changes coming into your lives. Allow them the freedom to be sad or angry. Encourage them to talk with others whom they respect and trust as they process their diagnosis. Seeing a mental health professional may be helpful. Emphasize to your loved one their significance in your life and in the lives of others. Help them navigate this new course in life and live each day to its fullest.

SHARING THE DIAGNOSIS WITH FAMILY AND CLOSE FRIENDS

We kept things to ourselves until we had a sure diagnosis. Early on we were told her symptoms might be associated with a thyroid problem, a medication she was taking, or a chemical imbalance.

One example of initiating this discussion with our immediate family was Jeanette's saying something off-base one day early in this journey. I decided to ask our daughter, Betsy, if she had noticed anything different about her mother. Betsy and I met that day, compared notes, and decided something was awry. That started the ball rolling to make another appointment with our primary care doctor, who then referred us to a neurologist.

Our family and close friends knew there was something not quite right with Jeanette but said nothing. When we were positive this was the journey we were on, we shared it with them.

The Alzheimer's Association offers the following insight on sharing the diagnosis:

> *Telling others about a diagnosis of Alzheimer's or dementia can be one of the most difficult steps for people diagnosed in the early stage and their care partners. There may be anxiety surrounding who to tell and concerns about social stigma.*
>
> *Sharing the diagnosis with others can open up new relationships and connections to people you did not realize were willing to support you. For others, hearing of the diagnosis may test relationships and some friends and family may react with denial, or pull away in ways that reflect their misconceptions about Alzheimer's disease.*
>
> *Yet, it can be empowering to share the diagnosis with others. Be open with friends and family about the changes that are taking place. Educate them on the disease and tell them how they can be supportive.*[1]

SHARING THE DIAGNOSIS BEYOND YOUR INNER CIRCLE

At some point it will be necessary and helpful to share your loved one's AD diagnosis with others beyond your inner circle of family and close friends. The following suggestions may be helpful to you:

- As your loved one may act normally in public, others may not realize anything is wrong with them. You need to inform others with whom your loved one interacts or from whom you need understanding and support.

- Others may not be surprised to learn your loved one has AD. They may tell you they had been noticing your loved one seemed fine on one occasion and on another occasion had difficulty.

- Be willing to talk about this new life journey. You do not have to share everything. However, a dialog with others may be more helpful than you can imagine.

- Talk with others who are on a similar journey so you can learn from each other.

- Never say anything you would not want your loved one to hear if they were cognizant of what you are saying.

Because I am a pastor and Jeanette had always been by my side, I knew I needed to inform my faith community so they could be knowledgeable of her condition and pray for her. I waited for a Sunday when Jeanette was unable to be present and shared our challenge. The church, and others who found out through word of mouth, were wonderfully supportive. They were gracious and tender with Jeanette. I found that net of love, encouragement, and support to be a lifeline in the years that followed.

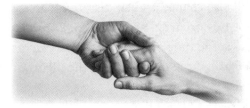

Scripture: "It was good of you to share in my troubles" (Philippians 4:14).

Prayer: *God, I am not good at this. Would You give me the words and the timing to share what needs to be shared, how much to share, and with whom?*

QUESTION #4:

WHAT SHOULD I
EXPECT TO HAPPEN?

Expect the unexpected. Your loved one's personality may be greatly altered. Their ability to interact with you in the way you expect will also change as their disease progresses.

An example of this occurred around 2015 when Jeanette and I were traveling by car to spend time in North Carolina. Out of the blue, Jeanette turned to me and said, "You cannot spend the night with me tonight."

"Why?" I asked.

"We're not married."

"Sure we are," I said. "Here's my wedding ring you gave me at Salem Baptist Church December 27, 1959."

"You can buy a ring anywhere and fake it," she responded. "Jim, I love you, but it just will not look right. What would Jesus think? What about our parents? It would invalidate everything we stand for. When we get married, you can spend the night with me."

Despite my efforts to persuade her otherwise, she was adamant about our not spending the night together. I gave up and did not mention it again. By the time we reached our destination she had forgotten her earlier declaration. Thankfully she did, as I was already thinking about having to sleep in the car!

INCREASING DIFFICULTY IN DOING NORMAL ROUTINE/ACTIVITIES

- You and your loved one's lives will change dramatically.

- Be prepared for a slow progression of dependence on you, the caregiver.

- Simple things like grooming and personal hygiene can become more difficult for your loved one.

- Your loved one will need assistance as they sometimes forget what a product or object is for and how to use it. (For example, Deb's dad needed help as he could no longer remember how to tie a necktie, which he enjoyed wearing to church or outings.)

- You will be doing things you have never done.

I was surprised at how quickly I had to learn to do many things I had never done. I started picking out Jeanette's clothes, assisting her in dressing and grooming, keeping the checkbook, shopping for groceries, making appointments, and accompanying her on every outside excursion.

One of the most challenging things for both of us was when she gave up driving. The doctor helped when he told her she should not drive because the medications might cause drowsiness and slow reactions. We soon found that out in our state, Florida, if one is being treated for memory loss and is taking certain medications, they are required to retake the driver's license exam. Jeanette did so, and, amazingly, she passed the test. The next day I let her drive a couple of blocks around our neighborhood. She navigated it well. When we got back to our house, she gave me the keys and never asked to drive again.

Driving gave her independence. Now she was dependent on others. This realization had tremendous emotional overtones to her already declining mental capabilities.

Deb's Experience:

I can remember my dad always taking care of me as a little girl. He was my protector, helper, and teacher. I learned so much about life from my dad. The roles reversed after he was diagnosed with Alzheimer's. I became his protector, helper, and teacher. I had to put things away that would harm him. I had to clean up messes he would make. I had to be his advocate and speak up for him, not only to protect him, but also to get the help that he so desperately needed. I had to help him remember how to do something his memory had forgotten, to coach him, and to show him how. He would use products incorrectly. He would put toothpaste in his hair or brush his teeth with the wrong product.

As the disease progressed, he no longer could be taught or reminded how to do something simple like brushing his teeth. He always needed help. I found myself combing his hair, brushing his teeth, helping him put on his shoes, helping him to bed, and even feeding him. While my heart broke in the moment of helping him, I also realized he needed me much like I had needed him when I was a little girl. The roles had reversed.

INCREASING DEPENDENCE ON THE CAREGIVER

- At first you will not realize the demand AD will take on you as the caregiver.

- You will be making all of your loved one's important decisions: medical, financial, palliative care, and end of life.

- While there may be windows of lucidity, these times will become rarer. All too soon the time will come when you will have to do the thinking for the both of you.

It is important to remember who the person was before the disease. Your heart will break on many occasions as you see your loved one slip away from the person you have known. Your loved one's personality will change. Most certainly, they will do and say things they never would have before getting this disease. They can be gripped with fear that causes them to accuse others of doing something wrong. They may get agitated and act out due to fear and frustration. Correcting or rebuking them in these situations will not be helpful as they are incapable of understanding what they are doing.

While you will not be able to predict what, when, or how your loved one will act or react throughout any given day, you as the caregiver can help your loved one by trying to maintain a calm attitude and response instead of reacting in a negative or harsh way. Never be confrontational but choose to redirect and coach them. Being proactive as much as possible will help you manage each situation with your loved one and keep your day from becoming overwhelming and stressful.

REMINDERS TO REVIEW:

- Learn to manage your expectations of caring for and dealing with your loved one and this disease.

- Do not treat this as a mental illness, but the disease of the brain: Alzheimer's disease.

- It is healthy to deal with your feelings of guilt—guilt over the times when you lose your patience and say things you wish you had not said or guilt when you feel you are not doing as much as you can or could.

- It's okay to cry. It's okay to laugh. Liken it to how you would respond if you were caring for a small child.

It is important how you approach and treat your loved one. They may look and act differently, but they are still the person you have always loved.

Deb's Experience:

As my dad got to the point he no longer knew us by name or that we were his family, I learned that when I approached him I needed to speak softly, call him "Dad," give him time to feel comfortable, and let me come closer to him. At that point, I could then give him a hug.

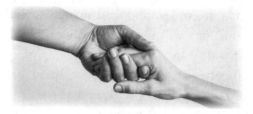

Scripture: "A time to weep and a time to laugh" (Ecclesiastes 3:4).

Prayer: *Lord, my emotions are running the gamut. They come and they go. Let me not linger too long in the highs and lows. Help me to sense Your Presence in them all.*

QUESTION #5:

WHO CAN HELP ME GET THROUGH THIS?

Throughout this journey of being a caregiver for your loved one, it is important to know there may be times you feel alone. Life as you have known it will begin to change. You will be called upon to make life-altering decisions without the usual input or encouragement of your loved one for whom you will now be responsible.

You are going to feel overwhelmed and alone as you tackle this challenge in its many facets. You should not attempt to go it alone. On your own, you will not be able to give your loved one the best care, nor will you be able to do what is best for your life and health.

Working with Your Family

It is important to work with your family. Meet with your family and share your challenges. There is greater agreement when a family works together.

If the AD patient is your parent and if you have siblings, seek to find ways to work together to do what is best for them. Be prepared to share the load, with each person using their giftedness or abilities to offer help as needed.

- Men and women, even siblings, can have differing opinions. Be respectful of each other in how you approach decisions that need to be made.

- Be willing to make hard decisions together.

- Extend grace to family members as each of you will deal with these kinds of challenges in different ways.

Deb's Experience:

I do not remember our family's sitting down and discussing who would do what to help with Dad's care. While I think this could and would have been extremely helpful, it just did not happen with our family. I feel that God directed my brother and me in assuming responsibilities according to our gifts and proximity to where Mom and Dad lived. This also freed Mom to love Dad in whatever time we had left with him.

Because my brother and I have a strong relationship, a mutual understanding of our differences, and complete trust in each other, we always remembered we promised our parents (long before our dad was diagnosed) we would never fight over their care, money, or possessions. I can say God gave us the strength and ability to honor our word to our parents.

We never made decisions without discussing it with each other to determine what would be best for our parents and honoring to them. We did not always agree. However, we respected each other and our parents enough that we worked together to find a solution. Our common goal was to make decisions that would be best for our loved one without causing problems for the family in the future.

My dad and brother, Steve, had been in business together. Steve lived only a mile from our parents. This made it easier for him to handle all the financial responsibilities that were necessary. He was familiar with how our dad did business and the way Dad would have handled certain situations. Their banking and other business matters were addressed in a similar manner and this was very helpful. Over the years, my brother learned how to be a great businessman from watching Dad. I trusted him to make the best decisions.

God equipped me to assume the role of dad's administrator with my responsibilities including his doctor appointments, caregiving, and other overseeing duties. Mom and I took notes on what was transpiring with Dad. I kept a log of the places to which Dad was admitted, as well as the meetings I had with the physicians and medical staff. This allowed us to more closely follow Dad's treatment, care, and the progression of the disease. It also prepared us to give information to the staff at the facility we were considering for Dad to receive the next level of care he needed. It became painful many times as I read the notes and saw how quickly this disease took the man we so deeply loved.

ENLISTING THE HELP OF CLOSE FRIENDS

You will want to try and do this all by yourself. Do not do that. Let others, who have the ability to do so, help you. As you identify specific needs, ask for help in those areas of care. If you do not have family to help share the load, ask someone whom you trust to come alongside you.

- When others want to help, it is good for them to know the needs and schedule of your loved one.

- Tell those who visit what to expect when they are around your loved one, so they will not be surprised. Short visits might be best for all involved.

- Ask your friends, church family, and support group to include you in their ongoing prayers. This will be your strength and help in this time of great need.

CONNECTING WITH SUPPORT GROUPS

The National Alliance for Caregiving estimates more than 65 million Americans care for a chronically disabled, ill, or senior family member or friend. Caring for someone with AD can present many challenges that can take its toll on the well-being and physical health of the caregiver, who often has to fight anxiety, sleep deprivation, exhaustion, isolation, depression. Finding a support group with whom to share stories, seek advice, exchange information, and from whom to get assistance can provide tremendous help for the caregiver.[1]

Call, go online, or ask others for help in finding a support group, such as Alzheimer's Association local support groups, Alzheimer's & Dementia Resource Center local support groups, Eldercare Locator, Family Caregiver Alliance, Memory People, and Veteran's Administration Caregiver Support. Local faith communities may also provide support groups as well.

- Be willing to be a part of a support group where you have the opportunity to surround yourself with people who have experienced what you are experiencing.

Seeking God's Help

This is a season of life when you may be sensing a need to seek help and strength beyond what others can. This is an opportunity for you to reach out to God and receive help like no other earthly assistance can provide.

- Prayer will connect you to God and be a source of peace. Hence, why we included a prayer and a passage of Scripture at the end of each chapter.

- You will find the faithful and loving God is always there whenever you seek Him and trust Him to get you through this challenge.

- God can help you learn to consider it a privilege to be honored with the opportunity to stand by your loved one who has stood by you.

Learning to Say "No"

While it is important to be respectful of differences with caregivers and family members, there will be times you must recognize that all help that is offered is not necessarily helpful.

- When others, whom have never been involved with caring for someone with memory loss, share their opinions, offer their advice or volunteer to help in caregiving, their help may not be beneficial. Learn to say "no."

- When the approach or care for your loved one is not done with dignity, it can be hurtful. Learn to say "no."

- When someone corrects or yells at your loved one instead of coaching or redirecting them, it can be hurtful. Learn to say "no."

- When someone talks to or about your loved one as if they cannot hear what is being said, it can be hurtful. Learn to say "no."

- When someone gives you legal or medical advice that is not trustworthy, it can take you down a wrong path, which is not helpful. Learn to say "no."

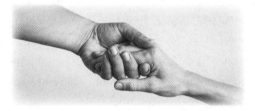

Scripture: "Carry each other's burdens" (Galatians 6:2).

Prayer: *God, I am so grateful for those good people You put into our lives to divide the load, and for You, above all, to lift the load.*

WHAT ROLES MUST I ASSUME TO PROTECT MY LOVED ONE?

T HE CAREGIVER OF an AD patient needs to stay one step ahead of the patient in order to keep them safe from him- or herself and the outside world. Much like the parent of a precocious young child, the AD patient can be deceptive in their words and appearance. The caregiver may be the only one who can correctly read the patient and anticipate outcomes of different situations. There are roles the caregiver must assume to protect their loved one.

LOOKING AFTER THEIR MEDICAL NEEDS

As the caregiver, you will become your loved one's medical advocate. It will fall upon you to know when your loved one needs to see the physician or specialist. You will need to inform all of your loved one's medical team of their AD diagnosis. This includes all medical professionals, including:

- Dental professionals

- Eye professionals

- Hearing professionals

- Therapists or psychologists

It is important for you to go to all your loved one's medical appointments. If you are not able to do so, then contact the medical professional about their current health status prior to the appointment or secure another informed caregiver or family member to take your loved one to the appointment.[1]

When accompanying the AD patient to see a medical provider, it will fall upon you to be the interpreter of their needs. Especially in the early stage of AD, your loved one will probably be able to deceive doctors who are not aware of the progression of their disease. At any given appointment, the patient may look healthy and act normal. Also, there is a difference in how a patient perceived their capabilities and the truth about their limitations. If medical care providers are not given the correct information, they can wrongly access the patient's needs and potential care or treatment.

You must help the doctor know what is truly transpiring in your loved one's life regarding matters of their physical and mental health. However, you must find a way in which to communicate the necessary information without embarrassing them or triggering anger in them by correcting them. Ideally, it would be better to inform the doctor or other providers in advance of the patient's inability to accurately access the patient and their needs.[2]

It will also fall upon you to keep track of your loved one's medical status, as well as the progressing symptoms of their disease. You will need to:

- Know their medical history, including all major illnesses and surgeries.

- Make sure their medical history and records are up to date.

- Bring an up-to-date list of all medications, as well as know all allergies to medications, anesthesia, et cetera.

- Bring your journal of changes in your loved one's health, reaction to medications prescribed for their disease, progression of their disease, including changes in their mood, behavior, abilities, eyesight, hearing, or mobility.

- Take notes and ask questions during appointments.

Storing your loved one's pertinent medical information in your cell phone or another readily accessible place will be important. This information should include:

- Medications

- Allergies

- Pertinent medical information

Always have important phone numbers on hand and stored in your cell phone, especially the phone numbers of:

- Family members to call in case of emergency

- Primary care physician

- Other medical professionals caring for your loved one

- Pharmacy

- Reminder: Call "911" in event of any medical emergency

Sooner, rather than later, begin investigating the availability, costs, and reviews of facilities that provide care for patients with AD. More information on this in later chapters of this book.

WATCHING OUT FOR
YOUR LOVED ONE AT HOME

As the caregiver, you will need to protect and watch out for your loved one with AD as one would do so for a young child. It is the caregiver's responsibility to keep the patient from getting harmed. It is important to make the home patient-friendly for your loved one:

- Add railings and fixture seating in the bathroom, including the toilet and shower.

- Make changes to rugs and carpets on which your loved one may trip.

- Give attention to steps and stairs. Install railings and keep stairways well lit.

- If possible, acquire a bed and chair(s) that are easy to get up and down.

- Be watchful in the kitchen. Pay attention to your loved one's access to the stove and microwave. Be on the alert for their leaving open refrigerator, freezer, dish washer, and stove doors. Take precautions with knives, as well as other potentially dangerous utensils and cooking tools.

- Be mindful in the laundry room: washer, dryer, iron, chemicals.

- Install locks on cabinets that contain anything potentially dangerous, such as toxic cleaning chemicals, medicine, and alcohol.

- Lock up or put away shop tools, knives, guns, outdoor chemicals, and other outdoor items that might cause harm.

- Store keys to your home, any locked cabinets, and all vehicles in a protected place.

- Take measures to keep doors, screens, and gates secure to keep patient from wandering off.

- Some alarm systems can be helpful in monitoring the opening of doors and windows.

- Having a baby monitor in the bedroom might be helpful.

- Installing security cameras indoors and outdoors may provide another level in keeping a watchful eye.

- Take precautions to protect your loved one from falling into swimming pool, if the home has one.

- Take fire safety precautions. Make sure carbon monoxide detectors, fire extinguishers, and smoke detectors are working. If your loved one with Alzheimer's smokes, always supervise smoking.

- Lower the temperature on the hot-water heater to prevent scalding or burns.

- Make sure the home is appropriately heated or cooled for the current weather conditions. For example, it is not uncommon for an elder to reach for a sweater or turn on the heat even though it might be unbearably hot outside.

- Remove mirrors that frighten your loved one.

We had to remove a large mirror in our hallway because Jeanette would see her reflection and not realize she was seeing herself. Thinking she was seeing someone else, she was either frightened or would start a conversation with her own image.

Guarding Valuables and Important Documents

Take measure to protect valuables (e.g., wallet, jewelry, important papers) your loved one might throw away, lose, or destroy.

There are two rings I regularly wore and cherished: my wedding band and my college ring. Sometimes I took them off because they cut into my fingers when I gripped golf clubs. I did so one day when I took a golf trip. When I returned home, I could not find my rings. Thinking I had left them in the shower at the golf club, I called to see if they had been turned in. No luck. I searched through my golf bag. No luck. Then I went through all my golf equipment. No luck. Then I searched throughout the house. No luck. I continued my search multiple times over a period of weeks. Still no luck. I was heartbroken over the loss of these legacy pieces. I finally gave up.

About four years later, I was going through some articles in the desk in my study at home. Behold, there were my rings! I apparently had left them on the top of our shower room chest of drawers—my usual spot for leaving things while I shower—and Jeanette must have decided to protect them for me by hiding them in my desk drawer. Lesson learned.

PROTECTING YOUR LOVED
ONE OUTSIDE THE HOME

To prevent your loved one from experiencing fear, getting lost, or incurring injury while outside the home, you or another caregiver should accompany them any time they leave the home. Also, a checklist of precautions to take while outside the home would include:

- Before leaving the home, make sure your loved one is appropriately (and completely) dressed for the weather conditions.

- Assuming your loved one is no longer driving a car and a caregiver is transporting them, it is imperative to follow the same safety precautions one would follow when leaving a child unattended in the car.

- Aid your loved one in walking safely to help prevent falling, getting lost, or wandering.

- Wandering away or getting lost from an unsecured home is a problem with some individuals with AD. The Silver Alert notification system, which sends area-wide alerts with information about missing senior adults, attests to this difficult issue. It may prove helpful for your loved one to wear a medical alert bracelet to help identify them, their AD, and other pertinent information.

- Busy, noisy, and unfamiliar places can intensify issues with your loved one.

- Encourage others you encounter to calmly approach your loved one. You may need to inform them your loved one has AD.

- When taking your loved one to be provided a service by a nail tech, hair stylist, or barber, inform them of their AD status. The same will be important if your loved one is being helped or fitted with a clothing purchase.

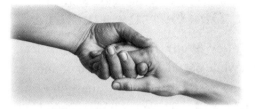

Scripture: "Lots of people claim to be loyal and loving, but where on earth can you find one?" (Proverbs 20:6, MSG).

Prayer: *Our Protector, my loved one needs me. As Your love and faithfulness is to us, let mine be for the one You have placed in my care.*

QUESTION #7:

WHAT FINANCIAL AND LEGAL PREPARATION DO I NEED TO MAKE?

C ARING FOR A loved one with AD takes a toll on families as they shoulder the financial burden of care.

- According to the U.S. Department of Health and Human Services, an estimated seven out of ten people age 65 and older will require some form of long-term care in their lifetime.[1]

- An annual report released by the Alzheimer's Association states that 83% of the help provided to care for a loved one with this disease comes from family members, friends, and other unpaid caregivers.[2]

- The total lifetime cost of care with dementia is estimated to be close to $342,000, with family care assuming 70% of that cost.[3]

EARLY FINANCIAL PLANNING

Establishing financial plans with and for your loved one after an AD diagnosis is essential. The earlier you can start a process of planning for your future is always a positive and proactive decision.

If you wait until your loved one is diagnosed with AD, it may be too late to make some of the necessary preparation or get the help they need for care. There will be necessary documents that need to be signed by your loved one when they are of sound mind. As the disease progresses, they will be incapable of making quick decisions. They may even resist or accuse you—someone they have always trusted—of taking their money.

- There's a greater risk that you will not have the finances necessary to provide the needed care if you wait until these things happen or progress rapidly.

- The decisions will fall on a family member or caregiver to make. This can create unnecessary hardships resulting in decisions which may not be in the best interest of your loved one.

Making plans for aging might not be a part of your thinking when young. However, we do not know if we will remain healthy as we age. The Alzheimer's Association projects that 1 in 3 seniors will die of Alzheimer's disease. Therefore, it would be wise to plan ahead should we or our loved ones need care.

EARLY LEGAL PLANNING

Make sure you seek legal counsel from those whom you trust or who come highly recommended. You may want to get counsel from an elder law attorney, as they specialize in laws and decisions pertinent to the aging. After receiving counsel from an attorney, you may decide to have some of following documents prepared for your loved one (and for you), get your loved one's signature on these, and store them in a safe place:

- **Last will and testament** outlines details of your loved one's wishes on how their estate is to be distributed at death and names an executor to manage the estate until its final distribution.

- **Durable power of attorney** allows your loved one to assign someone to manage their finances if they become incapable or otherwise unable to do it for themselves.

- **Living trust** makes funds and assets available more quickly than wills; allows assets in the trust to be distributed upon death or disability.

- **Living will** is one form of an advanced healthcare directive that specifies what actions should be taken for their health if they are no longer able to make their own decisions; e.g., life support.

- **DNR,** "do not resuscitate," is a healthcare directive that tells health care providers not to perform CPR.

- **Health care proxy** is a specific type of power of attorney in which your loved one authorizes someone to make medical decisions on their behalf if they are incapacitated.

There may be other legal or financial documents your attorney or tax accountant would recommend. It would be wise to get legal and financial advice on these and learn about ways to protect your other assets.

Preliminary funeral or burial plans should be discussed before your loved one can no longer offer input. You may decide to make purchases according to these decisions.

Organization and safe keeping of important documents will prove invaluable. Make a record of all financial and household accounts, including credit cards and electronic devices with usernames and passwords for all of them. This information should be available to the person authorized with the power of attorney and one other trusted person.

Ongoing Financial Burden

It has been reported that 35% of caregivers find it necessary to reduce their own working hours.[4] Some of the implications of the financial burden posed by AD include:

1. Facing possibility of loss of income

- Early onset AD can have a dramatic impact on finances.

- Government assistance is limited. Caregivers can lose government benefits if they work.

- Caregivers may lose income from their own jobs.

- Caregivers may be required to give up their careers by quitting their jobs or retiring early.

2. Facing possible need to divert income and savings

The average total annual expenditure to provide care to a loved one is estimated to be approximately $12,000[5] if the patient is able to live with the caregiver and does not require round-the-clock, outside assistance. Depending on the needs of your loved one and where you reside, it could be much more than this. This estimated amount does not include all medications and private care.

It also has been reported that nearly half of those caring for loved ones with AD have to cut back on their personal spending to cover caregiving expenses.

3. Facing potential financial jeopardy

- Loss of financial security

- Loss of savings

- Loss of home

4. Facing ever-increasing expenses in caregiving

In the early stages you will probably notice little change in expenses, but as the disease worsens, the financial bar will begin to rise. This probably will be seen in the following areas:

- Medical expenses (including the purchase of medications)

- Home modifications (e.g., extra handles, grips, and bars, especially in bathroom)

- Safety precautions (including locks and security alarms)

- Furniture adjustments (e.g., lower bed for easier accessibility)

- Additional caregivers

- Personal supplies (including diapers and lotions)

- Clothing needs

- Travel/transportation expenses (including trips to medical facilities and physicians)

There will be unexpected expenses throughout every stage of this disease. If your loved one stays home during the last stage, additional items for comfort and convenience may be required.

Deb's Experience:

Each person diagnosed with AD will have a unique story that can range from one extreme to another. One person's story may be caring for a loved one who is able to remain at home without other issues complicating the disease. While others, like my family, have twists and unexpected turns that cause caring for their loved one to become more difficult and more expensive.

As my dad was a tall, strong, and determined man, it made it harder to redirect, coach, and help him. This led to our family's not being able to care for him at home, as well as often prevented him from being admitted to facilities that were not adequately equipped to care for Alzheimer's patients with behavioral issues.

Each time my family needed to have him moved to a new facility, it was costly and accelerated his decline. We were at the mercy of each facility and their fees/costs as Dad was a private, paying patient. With each move, transportation by ambulance to other states was expensive. When a move was necessary, often there would not be an immediate place for him to be admitted. This meant he would be admitted to a geriatric psychiatric unit in a hospital that served as an in-between place for him to receive care until there was an opening in a facility. We also had to shoulder the costs of new medications, when prescribed, and an additional full-time nurse or aid, which was necessary for him.

---

5. Needing Day and Respite Care

There are often expenses for paying for respite care or private nursing care that potentially could evolve to paying for 24-hour care.

What is respite care?

Respite care is short-term relief for primary caregivers. It may be care for a few hours, days, or weeks. It may be provided at home or away from home at such places as adult daycare center, healthcare facilities, government programs, or through hospice.

What is the cost of respite care?

Respite care is not inexpensive. Services charge by the hour, number of days, or weeks. Most insurance plans do not cover these costs. You will be responsible for paying expenses not covered by insurance, government assistance, or other funding sources.

6. Needing Long-Term Care

There is always the possibility of an Alzheimer's patient's needing long-term care. The cost of such care can be expensive. At the time of our writing this book, the following were the estimates for long-term care:

- **Nursing Home Care**: The average cost of a year's care in a private, Medicare-certified, long-term nursing home room is $104,000.[6]

- **Home Care**: The average in-home care costs $49,920 a year for 40 hours of help per week.[7]

- **Assisted Living Care**: A year in a one-bedroom assisted living care facility averages $57,000 per year.[8]

7. Needing Palliative or Hospice Care

- *Palliative care* is specialized medical care focused on relieving the symptoms and stress associated with serious illnesses, such as AD. The goal is to improve quality of life for both the patient and family. Palliative care is provided by a specially trained team of doctors, nurses, and other specialists who work together with the patient's other doctors to provide an extra layer of support.

- *Hospice* is a type of healthcare that focuses on the palliative care of a terminally ill patient's pain and symptoms while attending to their emotional and spiritual needs. It can be an excellent resource for you in providing palliative care and guiding you in making the best plan for your loved one's care.

In the United States, the term *hospice* is largely defined by the practices of the Medicare system and other health insurance providers, which cover inpatient or at-home hospice care to terminally ill patients who are medically certified to have less than six months to live. Hospice is 100% covered by Medicare for all eligible patients, as well as by most Medicaid and commercial insurance plans.

If you are not sure if your loved one might be eligible to receive hospice care, contact hospice providers in your area for a free evaluation. If your loved one needs palliative care, check out and compare the different hospice providers to find the one with which you feel most comfortable. Hospice can be a blessing and gift to you and your family in the care and passing of your loved one.

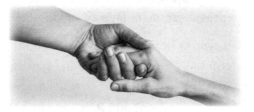

Scripture: "Plans are established by counsel; by wise guidance wage war" (Proverbs 20:18, ESV).

Prayer: *Counselor, show me the people who can give me wise counsel with integrity. Lead me not to delay, but get these important matters handled in a timely way.*

QUESTION #8:

WHAT CAN I DO TO PROLONG THE GOOD YEARS?

A DIAGNOSIS OF AD will cause the patient and those close to them to grasp at ways to hold on to a full and productive life for as long as possible. While the caregiver will be concerned about finding the best available treatment and care for their loved one with this debilitating disease, it is imperative for the caregiver to help the one with this disease to live their best life after the diagnosis and to find ways to improve their quality of life.

PROVIDING STIMULATING OPPORTUNITIES

- Provide opportunities such as music, art, or sports for your loved one, so they may continue to do what they love as long as the activity does not become too frustrating for them.

- Continue to provide opportunities for exercise such as walking, golfing, or taking exercise classes geared to their physical capabilities.

- If your loved one enjoys watching sporting events on television, you might want to enjoy this time of being together.

Deb's Experience:

Do not be surprised if they no longer want to do something they have always enjoyed. My dad loved watching sports on television. However, as his disease progressed, he suddenly thought these sports were stupid as he no longer understood the sports he once loved. His brain was no longer capable of processing what he was watching on television.

- Play their favorite genre of music, which can soothe your loved one. Sing. Move to the music. Dance.

- Enjoy vacation opportunities as long as possible.

Jeanette loved to travel, especially going on cruises. I took her on a cruise from Barcelona to Istanbul during the mid-stage of her Alzheimer's. She did well. She only got a little upset when navigating the airport in Rome, which can be nerve-wracking in the best of times.

We had a condo in North Carolina to which she loved going. I continued to take her there for three years after her diagnosis. As her illness worsened, and it became more problematic for her to travel, I sold it.

Jeanette loved art and painting. During her AD years she continued to work with crayons and colored pencils in adult coloring books. This continued until the late stages of her disease.

Jeanette was a talented pianist. She had been a finalist on the Original Ted Mack Amateur Hour when she was a teenager. She also had played the piano for worship services and sang in the church choir. She continued to play the piano after the onset of Alzheimer's.

Nearby neighbors, who were church friends, had a baby grand piano they would encourage Jeanette to play when we visited their home. When asked to play, Jeanette never refused. She would find a piece of music, sit upright at the piano, and begin to play.

She was able to play piano from early onset until the last year before she died. We recorded some of these moments. After her death, at the memorial service we included a final segment with her playing the song "Amazing Grace." When we recorded this, Jeanette got confused near the end of the stanza. It was there we stopped the video at her memorial service and had a bagpiper pick up where she left off—a special moment, indeed.[1]

Jeanette played golf through the early stages of Alzheimer's. Into the mid-stage she rode in the cart with me as I golfed. Being outdoors and with me seemed to have a calming effect, which I wish I had after some of my terrible shots!

Together we watched football, basketball, golf, and the Kentucky Derby. As a native Kentuckian, Jeanette always stood up and saluted when they played "My Old Kentucky Home," even in the late stage. She enjoyed eating popcorn, sitting beside me, and holding my hand as we watched these sporting events.

SOCIALIZING WITH FRIENDS AND FAMILY

- Keep your loved one socialized as long as possible, especially if they are living alone.

- Help arrange and facilitate opportunities for your loved one to continue to spend time with friends and family.

During Jeanette's illness, we were blessed with the births of several great-grandchildren. Whenever we would go to visit the new babies or they would come our home, Jeanette would hold them in her arms and smile. While she did not say much, she held them as naturally as she did with her own babies.

RELIVING MEMORIES

- There will be times when your loved one has "windows" of clearer thinking. Their memory will come and go as if a window is opened and then closed. Make the most of these times. The open windows will become more infrequent.

- Bring up old memories.

- Go through scrapbooks and old photos of days gone by and get them to tell you about the people they are seeing in photos. I found doing this to be incredibly rewarding. Jeanette loved looking at old photos of her family and special events. I would ask her about her elementary school days. She could name her principal, some of her teachers, and fellow students.

- Discuss old memories from early life, work, people they have known, places to which they have traveled over the years.

- Journal the recollections of your loved one. This can be a rewarding experience as you capture what surfaces from the springs of that amazing part of their brain.

- Do not miss the opportunity to make videos or recordings of your loved one as they reminisce. Do not be hesitant or embarrassed to capture these moments. This is part of their story.

Deb's Experience:

I am so glad I made videos of my dad while he was still alive. Two videos I treasure are of a time when my dad was playing guitar and another time when he was dancing with my mom (and leading her perfectly in beat with the music). He passed away two months after I shot the video of them dancing together.

Loving Them Well

- Show and express your love even on the most difficult days when nothing makes sense or seems impossible to bear.

Jeanette constantly told me she loved me. She would awaken me in the middle of the night to tell me she loved me. She would kiss me goodnight, and then want to kiss me again. She loved hugs and holding hands. She wanted to be cuddled. Usually quiet and not profusive with her words, she became the opposite during her Alzheimer's years. She still puckered her lips for a kiss from me until the last hours of her life.

I did everything I could to show and tell her I loved her. However, physical intimacy ceased after early stage as she began to confuse me with her father or brother. I did not want her (with her crippled mind) to feel she was being abused by people whom she deeply loved and trusted.

Christian worker, Vic Jacobson[2], whose wife fought dementia, expressed well the new normal for loving your spouse:

> *It can no longer be a search of the intellect, but has become a search of the heart, or should I say of the spirit. Language must depend less on words. Affectionate proximity is a language I believe she still understands. Nestling in my arms, holding hands across the table at teatime, laying her head on my shoulder as I pray for her. These are her dictionary of love.*

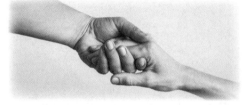

Scripture: "He will yet fill your mouth with laughter and your lips with shouts of joy" (Job 8:21).

Prayer: *Good Father, it is tough to find laughter and joy in this battle. However, with Your power I will do all I possibly can to bring laughter and joy to my loved one and, by Your grace, seize them when they come.*

SECTION II

WHEN THE DISEASE TAKES OVER

STAGE TWO SYMPTOMS OF ALZHEIMER'S DISEASE:

MODERATE OR MIDDLE STAGE

- This stage typically lasts the longest

- Symptoms from Stage One escalate in this stage

- Trouble performing activities (e.g., games, hobbies, driving, using a phone)

- Becoming less conversational (inability to remember to participate)

- Forgetting their current world (e.g., date, time, place, people)

- Becoming agitated more easily

- Making decisions is difficult (e.g., choosing weather-appropriate clothing)

- Getting lost more frequently

- Needing assistance and help

STAGE THREE SYMPTOMS OF ALZHEIMER'S DISEASE:

SEVERE OR LATE STAGE

- Symptoms from Stages One and Two continue to escalate
- Exhibiting severe cognitive decline
- Needing help around the clock
- Sleeping and eating habits drastically change
- Losing the ability to care for themselves (e.g., feeding, bathroom)
- No longer knowing their surroundings and how to survive without help
- Increasingly prone to falls, infections, and other illnesses

There is no way to know how long any one of the three stages of Alzheimer's will last with your loved one. Some research suggests the younger they are when they get Alzheimer's, the faster the disease progresses; the older, the slower. No matter which, it will seem as though time has stopped or you are in a time warp. Prepare the best you can for the long haul.

QUESTION #9:

HOW DO I TACKLE THE DAILY CARE OF MY LOVED ONE?

CARING FOR AN AD patient takes patience, forethought, and management. Your role as caregiver will evolve as the disease progresses. By the time the disease has progressed to stage two or three, you will not only be facilitating your loved one's medical care, overseeing their financial affairs, handling their legal matters, and protecting your loved one, but you will also be responsible for managing virtually all daily tasks.

Some individuals with AD may manifest signs of frustration or agitation when unable to perform a routine task. To reduce frustration, and help with the many challenges of successfully navigating your day, here are some tips:

ESTABLISHING DAILY ROUTINES

One of the most useful pieces of advice you might receive is to establish daily routines for your loved one. Some tasks, such as bathing and dressing, may be more easily accomplished earlier in the day when your loved one is rested and most alert.

Bathing and Grooming Routine

At the first stage of her disease, a shower was no problem for Jeanette. However, as the disease progressed, it become more problematic. Bathing was not an option, so I began to get in the shower with her. Later, our wonderful caregiver would shampoo her hair and wash her, usually twice a week. We did sponge baths the other days and times when needed.

- Make the shower time as brief as possible. Be organized. Have everything you will need on hand.

- Fear of water may become a big challenge as your loved one's vision and perception change. Showers can be scary as there seems to be a fear of the water cascading on the person.

- Some will resist bathing and showering, which makes it tough, if not impossible, on the caregiver if your loved one is larger and stronger than you. It can become dangerous for both of you.

- Hospice can be a wonderful resource in these situations. They will come several times a week (in the late stage) to help with bathing and other needs.

- You will need to help your loved one with brushing their teeth and grooming such as clipping nails, drying and fixing hair, and maybe even applying make-up.

- Use an electric razor for shaving.

Dressing Routine

As with bathing, establishing a dressing routine is helpful. Have your loved one dress at the same time of day each day, preferably earlier in the day.

- Encourage your loved one to dress him- or herself as long as possible. Sitting on a chair or on the edge of the bed usually is the best way to get this done.

- Limit clothing choices. To make decision-making easier, you may need to buy several of the same pieces of favored clothing.

- Clothes, shoes, and pajamas should be bought for comfort and ease in putting on and taking off. Avoid zippers and buttons. Select clothing with Velcro or elastic waists.

- If your loved one keeps trying to remove their clothing, there is adaptive and assisted clothing available.[1]

- In the later stages, the less changing the better, unless your loved one has soiled garments.

- As motor control diminishes, it will be more difficult for your loved one to help you when getting dressed.

- They may feel frustrated or even protest vigorously because they cannot move their arm or leg to help, which may also prove frustrating to you.

Eating Routine

Mealtimes can be challenging for you and your loved one. We found a few things to be helpful:

- Keep the environment as calm and free of distractions as possible.

- Offer a well-balanced diet. However, limit how many food choices you offer.

- Select foods that are more easily eaten and swallowed, especially if swallowing becomes more difficult as the disease progresses.

- Eventually, utensils will pose challenges. Spoons may be easier than forks.

I would try to include Jeanette in preparing for the meal, especially the evening meal. She loved being in the kitchen in her pre-Alzheimer's years, as well as during her illness. Up until the last stage of her illness, she enjoyed puttering around the kitchen. She would set the table, even though it was not always a conventional table setting. For example, she might put three spoons at one setting, which could be easily adjusted when she was not looking. She also enjoyed helping with limited preparation (e.g., stirring a fruit mix) and washing the dishes.

We always had a prayer of thanksgiving before we ate, which was something we had done all our lives. Often, I asked Jeanette to lead the prayer. Amazingly, she would always pray. Her prayers were usually focused on gratitude, although, occasionally they might wander to other items. When praying she would be lucid. It was if she was having a conversation with God.

Napping and Sleeping Routines

- Try to limit the number and duration of naps as much as possible, especially in the first two stages of the disease. This can help minimize the risk of your loved one's getting their days and nights confused.

- Establish a bedtime routine.

In the morning, Jeanette would awaken between 6:00 and 8:00 AM. I would give her breakfast. She would stay up for a while, take her morning meds, and go back to bed. She would awaken for lunch, take a brief nap, and then Sundowners Syndrome would hit. "Sundowning" will be discussed later in this chapter.

Jeanette would usually go to bed around 8:00 or 9:00 PM. She had been prescribed a cocktail of medications by her psychiatrist that I gave to her prior to our having our bedtime Bible reading and prayer, which was our sleep time routine. She usually slept all night, except for an occasional trip to the bathroom or to wander through the house.

We struggled with how much medication Jeanette should take. We did not want her to have too much and become a zombie or too little and be in a constant state of movement and agitation. We eventually felt comfortable with the pattern we established, although there was no perfect solution. You may have to experiment for a while to find the best routine for your loved one.

HANDLING DAILY CHALLENGES

Empathetic coaching can help assist your loved one when they are confused or agitated by simple decisions or tasks. Redirecting them is more productive than correcting them. Staying flexible with your routine, while trying to keep your loved one as content and calm as possible is the goal. Above all, treating your loved one with kindness and respect is paramount.

Communication

Communication is one of the major challenges of AD. Do not treat your loved one like a child. Instead, treat them with dignity and respect. Convey the following with your tone of voice:

- Talk lovingly to and with them. Tell them you love them often.

- Put yourself in their place. Show empathy for your loved one.

- Do not argue with or fuss at them.

- Do not correct them, especially in front of others.

- Do not say, "Do you remember?" They do not.

Confusion

Confusion is to be expected as you go about daily routines with your loved one.

- If your loved one does not recognize you, gently remind them who you are.

- Always remember your loved one is doing the best they can and would not be this way if they had a choice. There are ways to help without hurting.

- When asking your loved one to do something, establish good eye contact and offer simple, one-step instructions.

Simple routines could and did go awry with Jeanette and me. For example, once she put toothpaste on her toothbrush and proceeded to brush her hair with it. Another time she took lipstick and began marking her undergarments instead of putting it on her lips. During our mealtime one night she took salt and stirred it into her tea. These situations caused by Jeanette's being confused called for constant vigilance and gentle coaching.

Boredom

Your loved one may need simple tasks to help keep them busy when they become bored, which can occur at certain times of the day, especially in the late afternoon. These tasks need to be related to something they once enjoyed or did not mind doing. However, providing a task will not be productive if it causes them frustration.

Deb's Experience:

Because my dad enjoyed doing tasks with his hands, we had a basket with towels that he folded over and over again. Often, we would talk while he performed this busy work and I would thank him for his help. Simple tasks like this one often helped keep my dad from being bored and then wandering or getting into trouble.

Incontinence

If your loved one has incontinence and needs to wear adult diapers, please keep in mind they will need someone helping monitor and change them. Not attending to this need can cause other medical problems and irritations. They may also attempt to remedy their need in unconventional ways which can cause other issues.

- If you think about caring for toddler's bathroom challenges, it can help you anticipate what you need to do for your loved one.

- Limit intake of fluids in the evening.

- Taking your loved one to the restroom in public is a challenge. And it is a far greater challenge if that loved one is of the opposite sex.

Incontinence became a factor about the fifth year of Jeanette's illness. We purchased specially made diapers to keep at home, as well as in the car, in the event she had an accident while we were away from home. When she did have an accident, she would usually tell me. I checked regularly because a UTI (urinary tract infection) can be a problem. I always changed her diaper in the morning and before bed.

When we were in public and Jeanette needed to go to the restroom, I would ask another woman who was going in or coming out of the restroom to watch her, since I could not accompany her in the women's restroom. No one ever refused to help. They seemed glad to assist me when I explained her situation.

Sundowner's Syndrome

"Sundowning" or Sundowner's Syndrome refers to a state of confusion occurring in the late afternoon and spanning into the night. It can cause a variety of behaviors such as confusion, anxiety, aggression, or ignoring directions. Sundowning can lead to pacing or wandering.[2]

In our experience, sundowning would usually begin between 2:00 or 3:00 PM and continue for a couple of hours. With Jeanette, sundowning exhibited itself as restlessness, agitation, fearfulness, and hallucinations—the apparent perception of something not present. Jeanette's hallucinations included seeing men outside trying to get into the house to kill us, someone's being at the door, the school bus coming, her going to school, and her going to see her mom and dad at their house.

I found the best way to handle it was to redirect her. If she saw a "bad man," I would act like I was calling the police. If she was going to see her mom and dad, I would say, "They are not expecting us now, but I will call and tell them we will be there soon." Another thing that helped her when she was hallucinating was to give her half of a Xanax, which her doctor had prescribed. Even though it took about a half an hour before it took effect, it was helpful.

I discovered that if she had been out of her usual morning routine at the house—for example, if she went to church or the beauty salon—it made the sundowning worse. However, I decided it was better to keep her socialized and be prepared for a more difficult afternoon. This phenomenon seemed to lessen in the late stage of her journey with AD.

Some tips for reducing sundowning include:

- Trying to maintain a predictable routine for bedtime, walking, meals, and activities.

- Plan for activities and exposure to light during the day to encourage nighttime sleeplessness.

- Limit daytime napping.

- Reduce background noise, such as television. Play calming music.

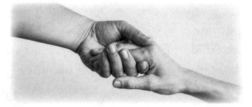

Scripture: "And your strength will equal your days" (Deuteronomy 33:25).

Prayer: *My Strength, I am counting on You. I often feel weak and inadequate. Out of my weakness, provide Your mighty strength. I rejoice in Your strength!*

QUESTION #10:

HOW DO I HANDLE NEGATIVE PERSONALITY CHANGES?

NEGATIVE PERSONALITY CHANGES often accompany the progression of this disease. The AD patient may display personality changes that are completely foreign to who he/she was before AD took over the brain. Experiencing and coping with drastic changes can be difficult and heart-breaking.

ERUPTING ANGER AND IMPULSIVITY

Sometimes, particularly in the middle stage of her disease, Jeanette would get angry if I did not let her go outside to "go home," "catch the bus," or "call the police to get that man who is trying to kill us." She would say, "You do not love me. If you did, you would do something about it." Even though I knew she did not mean it, the words still stung, especially when these incidents initially happened. It all was so foreign to what we had experienced in our relationship. I was at a loss to know how to best handle these outbursts.

> **Deb's Experience:**
>
> *My dad, too, expressed himself in uncharacteristic ways. On one occasion, when my parents were visiting and staying overnight with us in our home, my dad got confused and could not find the bathroom. This led to him wanting to leave immediately and*

go home. Dad told Mom that if they did not leave, he would jump off a bridge and kill himself. In response to his anger and impulsivity, my mom called my dad's physician, who had them return home and get his help.

As his disease progressed and his behavior became less remediable, my dad was moved to multiple facilities where he resided and received help to the degree those facilities could offer. While in residence away from his home, Dad would often get upset when he could not do what he thought he should be able to do. This would lead to his agitation as he did not know how to express himself. He could have these outbursts and become combative in any given moment. He never harmed or tried to hurt family members. However, there were times when Dad was in the care of medical facilities that his agitation was manifested through his actions.

Unfortunately, combative outbursts and inappropriate impulsivity are not all that uncommon with advanced AD patients. Their brains have been profoundly altered by their disease. Usually patients express aggression and agitation verbally. However, some may become physical. Contributing factors seem to be pain and discomfort, stress and confusion, as well as overstimulation—too much noise, clutter, or activity that overwhelms the patient.[1]

As I tried to learn how to navigate these episodes with Jeanette, I was given wise counsel by a physician friend. He summed up a helpful approach with the acronym T.A.D.A. This stands for: **T**olerate, **A**nticipate, **D**o not **A**ntagonize. It proved instrumental in my approach in coping and dealing with her.

GRIPPING DEPRESSION

Jeanette had dealt with depression for years and the Alzheimer's accentuated it. It revealed itself in her sleeping a lot, as well as her unhappy expressions when she was awake. Her doctor prescribed medications that somewhat alleviated these symptoms. This was more pronounced in the first two stages of her disease, particularly in stage one as she was coming to grips with this silent intruder, who was robbing her of everything she held dear.

Depression is very common among people with Alzheimer's, especially during the early and middle stages. As their disease progresses, it makes it increasingly difficult for them to articulate their sadness, hopelessness, and other feelings associated with depression. Deb's dad's depression was evidenced in his often being very sad, frequently crying, saying he was sorry for something he thought he had done wrong, and constantly asking Deb's mom to forgive him.

As the caregiver, if you see signs of depression, discuss these signs with your loved one's primary doctor, who is providing treatment for this disease. Getting a proper diagnosis and treatment may help your loved one improve his or her sense of well-being and functionality.[2]

DELUSIONAL BEHAVIOR AND HALLUCINATIONS

A delusion is a belief or altered reality that is persistently held, despite evidence to the contrary. Its most common form is schizophrenia. This behavior occurred with Jeanette in the middle stage and the early part of the last stage. Delusional behavior with her manifested itself usually as her believing one, two, or three men—bad guys who were walking, riding in a car, or standing outside our door—were trying to hurt or kill us. Her eyes would widen and in an agitated state, she would peer through the window or door. Her delusional state also caused her to hide things of value as she feared they would be stolen.

In its milder form, her delusions included the persistent fantasy that the school bus was coming, she was late for school, or she was going to see her mom and dad. She also thought the metallic plant on our fireplace was a live plant that needed constantly to be rearranged.

Responding to delusional behavior, as with many other symptoms of this illness, is best dealt with changing our attitudes and actions as the caregiver. Jeanne Murray Walter expressed it well:

> *I started letting go of my obsession of fixing my mother. I became like Sally in the Peanuts comic strip. I kept experiencing rude awakenings during the next several years—realities that I could not control everything. Over and over I grasped that*

whatever pilgrimage our family was on, I was not in charge of what the final destination would be or when we would get there.[3]

Deb's Experience:

When my dad was still being cared for at home, my mom could no longer sleep in the bed with him due to his hallucinations. He would kick and yell, which became a danger to my mom's being in the bed with him and possibly being hurt.

Coping Methods for this type of behavior include:

- Making an appointment to meet with your loved one's physician to see if there are medications that can help.

- Talking to your loved one in the reality they are in and not the one you think they need to be present in.

If they talk as if what happened years ago is current reality, that is where they are. You can join them in conversation in that place with them.

As another caregiver put it, "She erased the ghost of who her mother was and asked, 'Who are you now?'"[4]

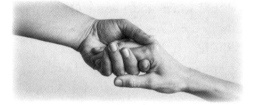

Scripture: Everyone should be quick to listen, slow to speak, and slow to become angry (James 1:19).

Prayer: *Gentle Shepherd, my loved one does and says things that wound me. Let me listen with discernment, subdue angry responses, and respond in the unfolding beauty of a gentle and quiet spirit. I want more of Your likeness in me, and less of me in me.*

QUESTION #11:

HOW MIGHT I IMPROVE MY LOVED ONE'S QUALITY OF LIFE?

A s you seek to help your loved one live the best life possible, you will want to try to keep him or her socialized, exercised, and stimulated. Providing opportunities to improve his or her quality of life can help both of you handle the daily patterns of managing this disease.

PROVIDE OPPORTUNITIES OUTSIDE THE HOME

It will prove beneficial for you and your loved one to get out of the house. Social interaction and activity are vital to handling this encroaching disease.

Exercising

If your loved one has exercised in the past, continue to do so as long as it is reasonable. You may find exercise increasingly difficult as the disease progresses. They will need more rest time and indicate this by telling you, "I'm tired" or "I want to go home."

Jeanette had always exercised, so we continued to follow her routine. Because of her weakening heart, fatigue became a factor we needed to manage. She also became less secure in her footing. Holding onto her as she exercised was a protective and comforting measure.

Dining out

"Do I take my loved one out for meals?" Yes, of course, you do! There is a tendency to keep them cloistered because of our fears of what they may say, how they might handle their food, or how they will deal with a bathroom visit. However, it is worth the effort for both of you.

I found that the wait staff in restaurants would make extra effort to ensure our meal experience was a good one. Some caregivers have chosen to print a business-type card to which they give the server. It simply states, "My loved one (wife, husband, mother, father...) has memory loss. Thank you for understanding and assisting us in making this a pleasant experience."

I always gave Jeanette a menu. She would look it over, hand it back to me, and either say nothing or respond, "Whatever you want is okay with me." I would then point out something and suggest, "Let's try this." Doing this kept it simple, alleviated pressure and gave her the dignity of doing what everyone else was doing.

Sometimes I had to cut up her food as handling the utensils became more problematic. Other times, she wanted to try to do it. I learned to go with the flow.

Getting out of the house

We tried to get out of the house as much as possible. Short rides to fun destinations were a regular part of our routine. Jeanette enjoyed going out for some of her favorite sweets: frozen yogurt, Italian ice, or Dairy Queen treats.

Jeanette also enjoyed getting manicures and pedicures. She never had a problem sitting for these. Likewise, getting her hair cut, shampooed, and styled were relaxing experiences for her. Happy to be getting groomed, she would sit patiently.

Often when she would model her new haircut for me, I would sing, "Here she comes, Miss America!" She always smiled when I did this.

I also took her to movies, the theatre, the Candlelight Processional at nearby Walt Disney World Resort, and the Singing Christmas Trees at our church. Two hours were about her limit at these events. Sometimes she would nudge me, indicating it was time to leave.

Sensitivity to your loved one's needs and limits is important. As times moves along, you will be able to discern their comfort levels as they usually cannot verbalize their desires. Observe and listen to your loved one as they will show you how to do what is best for them at the time.

Providing Opportunities at Home

It is not necessary to leave your home in order to improve and elevate your loved one's day. The following are some of the opportunities that our caregiving helpers and I provided Jeanette:

A. Entertainment

Singing and music were important in Jeanette's life. One of her caregivers, Arlicia, would play familiar religious and secular music from her laptop computer. Songs by John Denver, Johnny Cash, Nat King Cole, and the Gaithers were often played for Jeanette. "Tennessee Waltz," "Country Roads," "How Great Thou Art," "The Old Rugged Cross," and "Jesus Loves Me" were favorites played time and again. Jeanette and Alicia would sing along. I, too, would join them on occasion. She never got tired of this musical ritual, which was performed nearly every day. On her death bed, we played music our daughter, Kitty, had recorded until Jeanette went to heaven.

- Make entertainment choices that do not agitate your loved one.

- Play music from their favorite genres that are soothing to your loved one.

- Encourage your loved one to play a favorite instrument as long as they are able to do so.

B. Spiritual Practices

Church worship was always important to us. Until the later stages of the middle period of the disease, Jeanette was able to attend Sunday School in addition to going to the worship service. In her Sunday School class, she occasionally answered questions. In the worship services, she would have a friend sit with her if I was preaching that day. She sang the hymns from memory. If the pastor or teacher would ask us to open our Bibles, one of us would help Jeanette find the place in the Bible. Even though she could no longer read it, she would look at the Bible. After the worship service, she would greet people, even though she would not recognize them, and usually say, "God bless you." She was able to attend worship services until the very late stage of her disease. In fact, she was in a worship service the Sunday before she collapsed with heart failure.

In our home, I would read the Bible with her every night and pray with her. I would read certain Psalms and familiar passages, such as the "Sermon on the Mount" or the "Ten Commandments." Because Jeanette was raised in a Christian home and the Word of God was firmly embedded in her mind, I could quote Psalm 23, pause at certain places— like "The Lord is our ____ (Shepherd)"—and she could fill in the blank.

The Bible was a comfort and strength for her. Sometimes I would read aloud the devotional book *Jesus Calling* to her. I would ask her if she wanted to read the Bible or the book and she would either do it herself or say, "You do it."

We would pray together. Sometimes she would pray aloud. Her prayers were beautiful, trusting, and conversational. I wish now I had recorded her voice as she prayed some of sweetest prayers I have ever heard. One evening she prayed: "Lord Jesus, I love You. Thank You for this day, for going to church, for giving tithes, for [my brothers,] Bobby, Larry, and I going [to church], for our brothers and sisters, for my Jim, who is such a sweet man, for Your goodness to us, and for Your Holy Spirit. Help us. Lord Jesus, I love You. In Jesus' Name, Amen!" Then she added, "Thank You for all the good things You do for us."

Every evening after we prayed, I would tell her three things: "I love you. I am here for you. I've got your back." She would repeat each phrase back to me with some minor revision. She would usually respond, "I'll always love you." Sometimes when I would say, "I've got your back," she would teasingly reply, "I've got your front," and we would laugh. Then we would kiss goodnight. That was our routine for nearly every night throughout her illness.

Even though you may not recognize it, there are spiritual benefits your loved one will receive from the following spiritual practices:

- Singing together

- Reading/reciting the Bible together

- Praying together

- Worshipping together—for as long as they are able to do so

C. Touch

The importance of touch in our lives cannot be underestimated. It can calm our souls, elevate our mood, convey affection, and make a connection beyond words. In most situations, your loved one, like a child, will benefit from:

- Holding hands

- Rubbing feet or head

- Kissing (if appropriate)

Holding hands and putting my arm around Jeanette's shoulder were love touches and a serenity blanket to her. While watching television, sitting at church, or driving the car, I continually held her hand. If I was a little slow in taking her hand, she would reach for mine. When she would lie down for naps or at bedtime, she wanted me to lie beside her. Often during the night I could feel her hands touching me from the top of my head to my feet. While this could last for minutes, I never interrupted, because that touch represented my presence and security to her. She often would squeeze my hand, which she always did from our early courtship. This continued until a day or two before she left us.

Louise Penny, as she reflects on caregiving for her dementia-suffering husband, sums it up the best:[1]

> *I have promised myself that when he touches down, he'll be at home. Here. With me, holding his hand. Please, dear Lord, let that be one last promise I can keep.*

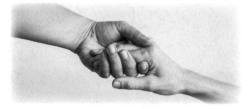

Scripture: "But Jesus came and touched them. He said, 'Get up, don't be afraid'" (Matthew 17:7).

Prayer: *Compassionate Jesus, let me be Your quiet voice and Your gentle touch to bring security and comfort to this special person so that fear must retreat.*

HOW DO I TAKE
CARE OF MYSELF?

CARING FOR A loved one with Alzheimer's can be overwhelming. A plan for taking care of yourself to be put into place earlier than you may think is needed. Do not neglect yourself. You must attend to your physical, mental, and spiritual needs as you will face more hard, sad, and emotional days than you ever thought you could handle. The best thing you can do for your loved one is to stay physically, emotionally, and spiritually strong.

You will have to deal with isolation and feelings of depression, which will be exasperated by your physical exhaustion from lack of sleep and providing care 24/7. Plus, your loved one may shadow you—follow you constantly—as you are their last touch with reality.

RECOGNIZING THE SYMPTOMS
OF CAREGIVER STRESS

Often, the primary caregiver is forgotten and ends up needing to care for themselves. The Alzheimer's Association has provided the following **Caregiver Stress-Check:**[1]

- **Denial** about the disease and its effect on the person who has been diagnosed. *I know Mom is going to get better.*

- **Anger** at the person with Alzheimer's or frustration that he or she can't do the things they used to be able to do. *He knows how to get dressed—he's just being stubborn.*

- **Social withdrawal** from friends and activities that used to make you feel good. *I don't care about visiting with the neighbors anymore.*

- **Anxiety** about the future and facing another day. *What happens when he needs more care than I can provide?*

- **Depression** that breaks your spirit and affects your ability to cope. *I just don't care anymore.*

- **Exhaustion** that makes it nearly impossible to complete necessary daily tasks. *I'm too tired for this.*

- **Sleeplessness** caused by a never-ending list of concerns. *What if she wanders out of the house or falls and hurts herself?*

- **Irritability** that leads to moodiness and triggers negative responses and actions. *Leave me alone!*

- **Lack of concentration** that makes it difficult to perform familiar tasks. *I was so busy I forgot my appointment.*

- **Health problems** that begin to take a mental and physical toll. *I can't remember the last time I felt good.*

All these symptoms in the caregiver's life need to be addressed by the caregiver and their doctor. It is critical to address these as they can cause one's physical and mental health to decline.

An often-cited Stanford University study found that 40% of caregivers die from stress-related disorders before the patient.[2] This study goes on to say caregivers have a 63% higher mortality rate than non-caregivers.

DEALING WITH CAREGIVER STRESS

The following guidelines are aimed at wellness for the caregiver:

- Visit your healthcare providers for regular check-ups to help with any physical and mental issues you may be experiencing.

- Remember that you are not alone. Let others help you.

- Get out. Take periodic breaks from caregiving. Spend time doing something for yourself and with others. While you might feel guilty leaving your loved one for short periods of times, it is necessary.

Deb's Experience:

As my brother and I helped care for Dad, we made sure Mom knew we were coming to give her a break. We encouraged her to get out of the house and make plans to do things she enjoyed. This proved to help Mom stay mentally and emotionally healthy during our care for Dad.

- Exercise. Get moving. Do not neglect exercise as it is an important part of staying healthy. It can also help with stress relief, disease prevention, and an overall feeling of wellness. Take friends and family members up on their offers to help you so you can make time to exercise, even if it is just for a short period of time. Thirty minutes per day can make a huge difference in your life.

- Eat well. Make healthy eating a priority. This will be good for you and your loved one.

- Be encouraged. You will get through this. Count every day as a success.

A pastor friend, Rev. Ray Lee, who lost his wife to dementia penned these words to me after her death:

It was a privilege to care for one who had shared my life for all those long years. Nevertheless, I did not realize the toll it would take on my physical and emotional strength. When the choice came between taking care of her desires and needs or my well-being, I willingly acquiesced to her. To be a caregiver twenty-four hours a day is not easy by any means.

People mean well when they say to a caregiver, "You should take care of yourself," but unless [they] have walked that road they cannot begin to understand how difficult this may be. However, [for a caregiver] to not understand how to care for one's health or fail to do so may have serious consequences later, as I was to discover.

Rev. Ray Lee, ended up in the emergency room and in the hospital for a five-day stay after his wife's death. This was followed by three weeks of home therapy. He was exhausted from extreme dehydration and physical fatigue.

- Live life one day at a time.

I learned I must live life a day at a time. An example of how I wrapped my mind around this necessary, new existence had to do with my preparation of the pill box containers for Jeanette's medications. Each container had seven days on one side and seven nights on the other. One day as I was filling the containers, the thought ran through my mind that my life was being measured by pills: one day, one night, one week at a time.

My therapy became a round of golf with friends, an occasional movie, or a meal with friends. After Jeanette fell asleep, I could sit on the back porch to relax, meditate, and plan. However, I always kept a sensitive ear to her voice. If she awoke and came to the porch, I would invite her to sit with me. When she did, she usually positioned herself where she could see me.

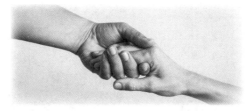

Scripture: "He gives strength to the weary and increases the power of the weak...Those who hope in the Lord will renew their strength. They will soar on wings like eagles; they will run and not grow weary, they will walk and not be faint" (Isaiah 40:29, 31).

Prayer: *My Eternal Rest, when You walked among us You took some time apart. Grant me the wisdom to do the same and not feel guilty about it.*

WHAT SHOULD I CONSIDER IF CONTEMPLATING A LONG-TERM CARE FACILITY?

W HILE I WAS able to provide all the caregiving for Jeanette at our home, many others, like Deb, have to make the tough decision about seeking long-term care. You may be someone who is facing difficult choices you never thought you would have to make. Your loved one may need care that is beyond what you can provide at home. Your home may no longer be the safest place for your loved one to live.

EVALUATING YOUR AND YOUR LOVED ONE'S NEEDS

- Your health may be deteriorating as you care for your loved one. You may need help so that you can stay mentally, physically, and emotionally healthy.

- Explore the resources available to meet the needs of your loved one and how they will work with your insurance and budget. For example, if your loved one has served in the military, are they in the system to be able to receive care in a veteran's facility?

- Removing the phrase, *"I put my loved one in a home"* and replacing it with, *"I need to find a safe place for my loved one to live and get the best care"* will help you deal with this difficult decision and affirm that you have done everything possible to care for them at home.

- It can be difficult to make this decision. However, realize that you may have gotten to the point that it is necessary so that your loved one can get the best care and you can take care of yourself.

Deb's Experience:

Home has always been special to our family as we always lived in a small town. Home was where we shared love with a multitude of extended family members, friends from our hometown, and our church family. Our home was one that said "You are welcomed here." Our home exhibited the finest hospitality by my Southern born-and-bred-mom.

My dad loved home. I think because he did not grow up having a place that looked or felt like home, he wanted our home to be a special place for family and friends. When Dad was beginning to have memory issues that were quickly progressing, we were determined do our best to keep him in the home he loved for as long as we could.

We did our best to research and learn about our best options for his optimal care. After doing so, we felt we had a plan in place. We took my parents' master bedroom and created a safe place for Dad to live. We removed everything in the bedroom that could be of danger—mirrors, extra furniture, et cetera—and created a comfortable place for him in their spacious bedroom with a sitting area and master bathroom.

This set-up only proved to be the best place for my dad during the first year. Dad was strong and always trying to get out and get away, no matter where he was, even when at home. It was a constant challenge to keep him safe at home. It worked for a while; however, with his mobility and physical strength, it became too much for us to monitor.

To make matters more challenging, one day Dad began having a horrific headache that would not go away. My brother, Steve, took him to the hospital, where Dad was admitted. They found my dad had experienced a significate stroke. His Alzheimer's progressed more quickly after the stroke. It became obvious we would not be able to continue the living-at-home situation long-term and so we started looking for the next option for his care.

My mother also needed greater assistance with my dad. As I lived two hours away, it became necessary for me to travel to my parents' home to stay during the week and for my brother and sister-in-law to stay with Mom to help on the weekends. During that time, we had the support of our local hospice facility located a few miles from my parents' home. They had a beautiful wing called Shepherd's Cove, where my day stayed a few times in their respite care to give us all a break. This was a great resource.

The day came when hospice told us it was getting too dangerous for us to keep Dad at home. Dad was a strong, fit, and outwardly healthy man. As his brain was being taken over by the disease, his behavior drastically changed. He tore wallpaper off the wall, almost completely took apart a Lazy Boy chair, and almost pulled the toilet from the floor in the bathroom. He did not know what any of these objects were, much less how to use them. Even though his own family was caring for him daily, he did not know our names, although I believe with all my heart, he knew we were special to him in his home.

Dad never hurt or even tried to hurt any of us. He never cursed or did anything at home that caused us to fear him. However, he did cause us great mental anguish and exhaustion. One of those trying times happened one night when my brother and his wife were staying with Mom. My brother kept hearing a noise across the hall. He went into the room and found our dad in the adjoining bathroom. Dad was trying unsuccessfully to open the window. Dad saw my brother, did not know who he was, and said, "I'm sure glad you showed up. I need you to help me get out of this place!"

Of course, my brother talked to him and helped him get back in bed. We still laugh about this crazy, middle-of-the-night encounter. We faced a number of these occasions and chose to approach them with love and laughter to help lighten the load and move on. However, these sorts of episodes helped us know for certain it was time to relocate Dad to a place where he could be safe and get the next level of care he needed.

CHOOSING THE RIGHT LONG-CARE FACILITY

Do your homework and research the closest facilities that can best meet the needs of your loved one. Make an appointment with each facility to get a tour and talk with their team.

Talk to current residents and their families during the tour. Observe the appearance and hygiene of the residents. Note the odor of the building. Are there patients who are screaming or hollering?

View rooms or apartments of current residents with their permission. Resident's positive or negative attitude is an indication of their social interaction with staff and other residents.

Make a point to tour the facility during mealtime. Tour the dining room and observe the meals served. Tour activities in progress. There should be posted a calendar of activities for the month.

Joey Keen, the Director of Operations for Senior Living Management Corporation—a corporation involved in all aspects of senior housing and retirement living in Florida, Georgia, and Louisiana—advises potential residents and caregivers to arrive at potential facilities for unannounced tours. She lives by the mantra "do not expect if you do not inspect." She also provided the list of questions below. She advised that the answers to these questions should confirmed before making any decisions. Most can be confirmed by viewing regulatory websites that each state offers.

QUESTIONS TO ASK WHEN INTERVIEWING POTENTIAL FACILITIES

1. What level of care does the community provide?

2. What type of training has the staff received?

3. What is the monthly rate for housing and care? What services does that rate include?

4. Are rooms private or semi-private? How do prices vary for each?

5. What level of personal assistance can residents expect?

6. What is the policy for handling medical emergencies?

7. How is the community secured? Are patients and their personal items safe?

8. What meals are provided? Are special dietary requests, such as kosher meals, accommodated?

9. How often are housekeeping and laundry service provided?

10. What programs (exercise, physical therapy, social and other activities) does the facility offer?

11. Does the facility accommodate special care needs, such as diabetic care, mobility issues, physical aggressiveness, or wandering?

12. Are residents grouped by cognitive level?

13. What is the ratio of staff to residents during the day/night?

14. How does the facility communicate with families about a resident's well-being?

15. What is the discharge policy?

When touring a facility for a loved one who has symptoms of dementia or Alzheimer's, it is imperative to tour the memory care unit. Focus on the same criteria listed above. Other questions you will want to address include:

1. What is the ratio of certified nursing assistants (CNAs) to registered nurses (RNs) or licensed practical nurses (LPNs)?

2. How often are patients checked on by the staff?

3. Are naps scheduled?

4. Are patients awakened for their meals?

5. Are they monitored in bed at night? Can they wander and possibly fall?

In addition to doing your research, interviewing staff, and visiting potential facilities, you must allow your instincts to guide you. Some places may not be a good fit for your loved one. You should be able to discern what is right.

Finally, as you are considering your options and comparing facilities, it is important to obtain via contract the cost for additional services that may be required at a given facility.

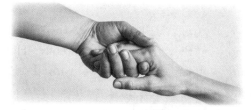

Scripture: "You hold me by my right hand. You guide me with Your counsel" (Psalm 73:23–24).

Prayer: *Sovereign God, I am bewildered at the choices and decisions I must make. You are not. You promised Your counsel and Your guidance. I believe You and will act in confidence—not leaning on my fears but being held securely in Your big hand.*

QUESTION #14:

HOW SHOULD I WORK WITH A FACILITY'S STAFF TO ASSURE BEST CARE?

A LL LONG-TERM CARE facilities are not the same in how they are staffed and what they are committed to offer. However, there are some things you can do to make your loved one's experience as positive as possible while residing in a facility. The following are some ideas for how you might accomplish this.

STAY INVOLVED IN THEIR CARE

Make the decision to remain involved in your loved one's care as much as possible. This is vital.

- Help groom and feed your loved one as you are able to do so.

- Take your loved one for walks by foot or wheelchair.

- Talk lovingly to and with your loved one.

- Find joy in times that you can laugh to help ease the pain of your loved one's dark and lonely existence.

- Enjoy music: listening or singing.

- Follow through on the desires expressed by your loved one as much as possible.

- For people of faith, read Scripture and pray when able to do so.

Deb's Experience:

Mom often read Scripture to Dad and asked him to repeat certain verses. She would pray for him. These practices helped bring calm to Dad's storm with this disease.

WORK WITH THE STAFF AND MEDICAL TEAM

- Meet with the medical team where your loved one will be residing to discuss a plan.

- Get to know the medical team and the shifts that they work. Learn their names. Let them get to know you and the other caregivers.

- Show up often and unexpected at your loved one's new residence.

- Ask questions of the staff and caregivers (without interrogating or accusing).

- Build relationships with the caregivers.

- Let the caregivers know how much you love the person for whom they are caring.

- Document times when you recognize or see things that are not right.

- If the place is not right for your loved one, then make changes to get them moved to another facility.

Deb's Experience:

My dad was in and out of multiple facilities during the last two years of his life. He spent time in hospitals, respite care, nursing homes, geriatric psychiatric units, a state mental hospital, and a hospice care facility. Most of these places were often not staffed or equipped to care for his compound issues and needs. He was physically strong and very mobile with advanced Alzheimer's disease. This created combative behavioral issues, which made him a troublesome patient anywhere that he received care.

I remember my mom and I having this disease described to us in the following way:

"Imagine if you were to be captured with only what you have on and what you have with you. You are blindfolded and taken in a helicopter to a foreign country. You are dropped into this unknown country, only to find out that you do not know where you are, the language that is spoken, or the people who are around you. Nothing makes sense. You are fearful and confused, because you cannot understand where you are, how you got there, how to survive, or how to get out."

This was a powerful explanation of an Alzheimer patient's world that will forever be etched into my memory.

My goal was always to find a facility that first and foremost could and would care for my dad with dignity while keeping him safe and meeting his needs. I also wanted to find a place as close to home as possible. This was important not only to my mom, brother, and me, but also to our family who lived close enough to visit. We were dedicated to visiting almost every day, and we remained very involved in the care he received.

Most places where my dad was cared for, we were thankful for how he was being treated and having his needs met. However, the day came when we could not find a place to care for him. We had exhausted all possibilities as he had already been to most of the facilities in our area. At this juncture, our doctor met with us and told us there was a mental institution where he could receive care. He would have to be "committed," which meant my mom would have to sign papers to legally have him committed to this facility. This was our last resort.

This was the day when we thought we would not make it. We struggled with the thoughts: "How could we do this? Where else was there to go?" Our hearts broke that day as my mom and I held each other and cried. This was not in our plans for Dad to have this as part of his Alzheimer's journey. However, we were at the end of our rope. There was no other facility that would or could take care of him. We certainly did not see this coming but found this was another part of the uncertainty of the disease.

One day when my husband and I visited Dad, I noticed bruising on several parts of his body. I knelt beside the wheelchair and said, "Daddy, what happened to you?" At this stage of his disease, Dad was basically nonverbal. However, he quickly answered, "They really worked me over." I wept. I looked up at my husband with a look that said, "Did you hear that? Can you believe they would mistreat my dad?" My dad could no longer really communicate, but he did in that moment. He had just said something that made sense and let me know what I had hoped was not true.

I began to take notes of each visit and document what I observed. I requested a meeting with the medical staff. I was heartbroken due to the lack of care or response from that meeting. My mission became to get him out of there.

With the help of several medical professionals and strong determination, we were able to locate a new place for my dad. It took several weeks, but God provided a facility where dad had not been, and we were able to get him admitted (not committed). This move was an answer to our prayers like none other!

Sometimes your best plans may get derailed. You may have to make decisions you never thought you would have to make.

If necessary, be willing to find another place to relocate your loved one. Keep in mind that each time a person with memory issues is moved and relocated to a new facility, it causes greater regression and adjustments as they are once again in another unfamiliar place.

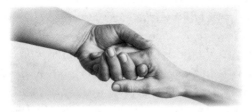

Scripture: "But in everything, by prayer and petition, with thanksgiving, present your requests to God" (Philippians 4:6).

Prayer: *Wonderful Counselor, show me how to be a team player with those I have entrusted to give the best of care to the one whom I have placed in their hands. May they respond by giving their best to us.*

QUESTION #15:

HOW SHOULD I EXPECT CARE FACILITIES TO HANDLE BEHAVIORAL CHALLENGES?

FOR THOSE WHO have experienced difficulty in getting the right kind of compassionate, excellent care for their loved one while in a care facility, and want to know what level of care should be expected, Deb has written this chapter with the contribution of invaluable insights from Annette Marlar, the Director of Medical Service in the Memory Care Residence of Job's Way at Kirby Pine Estates.

EXPERIENCING BEWILDERMENT WITH HEALTHCARE SYSTEM

My dad had numerous caregivers in multiple facilities during the last two years of his life and I am grateful for these people. However, I will forever feel indebted to Annette Marlar and her team at the Memory Care Residence of Job's Way in Memphis, Tennessee. This was the last facility where Dad lived. It was there our family had the privilege of observing and learning from a team of caregivers that sought to continue to learn from their patients the best way to provide individual care and treatment. Their example of striving to discover and implement the most informed care for individuals who are struggling with memory loss left such a lasting impression on my family and me. As such, I want to share our experience with you to encourage you with regard to the healthcare system and an exceptional approach available for caring for someone with AD.

While talking with Annette on our initial phone conversation about my dad, she recalled: "I quickly realized I was talking to a daughter who was bewildered by the healthcare system and at a crossroads of not knowing what to do to help her dad. I could hear the intensity in her voice as she described the trauma her dad had been through since he had reached the point where he could no longer safely be cared for at home."

In the previous twenty months my dad had been in four nursing homes and five Geri-psych units in two states and no one wanted to take him. However, Annette and her team gave me hope. Soon God provided another option for my dad through this remarkable team. Job's Way was to be his new home with their incredible staff who would provide the best, break-through care for him.

Annette helped me understand there are things you can do to help with the transition into a new home for your loved one:

- Once you find a facility that will be able to care for your loved one and meet their needs, you will want to ask for a meeting with the healthcare team to discuss a personal plan of care.

- You will then want to meet and work with the healthcare team to provide a history of how your loved one lived their life before and after their diagnosis with Alzheimer's.

- You will want to provide a description of your loved one's physical and behavioral lifestyle. It is crucial for you to partner with them to provide this history as it will give a framework for their 24/7 approach to care. The holistic approach is about adapting to the patient's needs.

Further notes from Deb:

For you to fully understand my dad's journey during his short stay at Job's Way, I want to discuss his first forty-eight hours there and how this team of caregivers approached his care. While the team was aware of his activity and agitation level, as well as his fast and steady pace in walking, they did not anticipate he would spend his first 21.5 hours walking with only brief stops to eat, hydrate, clean up, change his briefs, and allow them to assess his vital signs. As a staff, they came up with a plan to make sure he was safe and to have staff members walk beside him and change their shifts every hour.

Finally, on the third day, Dad went to sleep sitting straight up on the sofa. My thoughts quickly took me to other facilities where he had been and how I would often find him strapped to a chair or sedated. While my heart broke to think he was trying so hard to "get somewhere"—probably trying to go home, my heart also felt gratitude for this amazing team of caregivers who were willing to literally walk beside him. I realized the importance of his feeling safe.

Expecting the Best Care for Your Loved One

The following are some of Annette Marlar's insights that she has gleaned over thirty-five years of learning from the residents in her care who had Alzheimer's.

1. As human beings, our behavior is purposeful. Keep this in mind throughout your personal situations in working with a person who has Alzheimer's.

2. Dementia of the Alzheimer's Type does not define a person, but it is a part of the present of who he is and will become.

3. The person also has a personal lifestyle, personality traits, and a uniqueness that expresses who he is and the view of who he is in a mirrorless world.

4. The person is probably coping with co-existing diseases that can certainly contribute to how he is coping with Alzheimer's.

5. The person is aging and is coping with the aging process that can affect him physically, mentally, and emotionally.

6. There are three keys to caregiving that influence the decisions and actions of the caregiver. They are:

    (A) Anticipate the person's needs both scheduled and unscheduled.

    (B) Give the person his space.

    (C) The ultimate key: Do not provoke the person.

7. Have a Plan A, B, C, D, and so forth. As the moment changes, so can the person who has Alzheimer's. As the caregiver learns to adapt, the art of compassion takes flight and is demonstrated through knowledge, skill, insight, and empathy.

8. Be an investigator of the person's lifestyle before and as Alzheimer's progresses.

9. Labeling a person who is involved in a behavioral incident or event often can be one of the most impactful documentation errors healthcare providers can do, because that labeling probably will never be removed from the medical record. The important question is: *WHY did this situation occur?*

10. Caregivers can be right at the wrong time. Ask yourself if it is worth it to correct the person with Alzheimer's who thinks differently from you. If the person is safe, let the opinion or the procedure wait.

11. Get to know the whole person before you get to the care planning for the whole person.

12. The patient who has Alzheimer's often stays in a survival mode until he feels safe. He will probably act out in one or more of these ways: Fight, Flight, or Freeze. A good caregiver has the goal of providing a safe place where survival is not moment to moment.

Deb's Experience:

In his last night at Job's Way, Dad would not sleep in his bed unless someone was in the bed beside him. Once again, the team met his needs when they observed he was afraid and would not let him sleep in his bed alone. Annette remembers, "He slept in his bed under the cover and a staff member laid on top of the cover by him. Another staff member sat in a chair at the end of the bed while Ray slept. That night, he slept all night and even snored several times. He was tired and his body was exhausted." Was this an orthodox option? Maybe or maybe not. Annette remembers being told that none of the staff had a problem doing this because they were the ones who knew him well, had taken care of his many needs, and had devised this option so my dad could sleep.

Annette shared, "Our staff learned much from our time with Deb's father, Ray. He challenged us to become a better staff and realize how to journey into our personal beliefs about caring for someone with Alzheimer's. Little did we know we would literally walk beside him as he was trying to find his own path. Someone has said the best way to find yourself is to lose yourself in the service of others. That is what we had the honor to do with Ray."

You can see how invaluable it is to find the best facility for your loved one. In seeking to do this, meet with the healthcare team to learn their approach and willingness to provide optimal, compassionate care for your loved one.

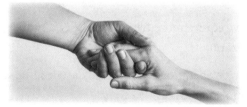

Scripture: "And my God will meet all your needs according to His glorious riches in Christ Jesus" (Philippians 4:19).

Prayer: *God of grace and mercy, grant those who daily seek to assist my loved one with all they need to give compassionate care, even when my loved one's behavior is difficult.*

QUESTION #16:

WHAT MIGHT I EXPECT WHEN THE END IS NEAR?

Y̲OU MAY OR may not be certain the end is near. An AD guide with information regarding what to expect at each stage might be helpful. Your physician(s), as well as hospice, can also help you know what to expect and when the end is near.

RECOGNIZING THE SIGNS

- Their sleeping habits may have changed.

- Their communication skills may have changed as some will speak less.

- Their eating habits may have changed.

- They may require more trips to the ER or more hospitalizations.

- They may be spending most of the day sleeping in bed or in a comfortable chair.

- They have started feeling weaker or more tired.

- They have experienced shortness of breath, even when resting.

- They may have fallen several times over recent months.

- They may need more assistance with daily routine, as well as getting up and down.

- Some experience weight loss.

Taking Necessary Action

- Your loved one's needs will be different. Being aware of these changes will help you provide the best care for them. You will need help from others now more than ever.

- The patient's doctor will advise when it is time to shift to hospice care. This care will make the patient as comfortable as possible, by managing the patient's pain and other distressing symptoms. Hospice will provide much help for your loved one, as well as for you as you try to understand what is transpiring and how you should respond.

- When you see your loved one's health is rapidly declining and death is imminent, it is a good time to talk with hospice, your pastor or counselor, and family members about the decisions that will need to be made when they pass.

- Among practical considerations is to handle some necessary things prior to your loved one's passing. For example, write the obituary, as much as possible, ahead of time. You can add the remaining details after your loved one passes. In lieu of flowers, you may want to go ahead and determine to whom memorial gifts, (e.g., contribution to a charity), may be given. You will also need the address where memorial gifts may be sent.

Recognizing Possible Near-Death Experiences

Near the end, Jeanette had been home six days since her emergency visit to the hospital. She mostly rested, sporadically ate light foods, occasionally communicated when asked simple sentences or to say "thank you" or "I love you." I really thought she was going to regain her strength so I was shocked on that Tuesday when I was told by the lead nurse, "She's dying." The words were so chilling, and yet so matter of fact.

Our constant vigil continued as we lingered by her bedside and watched her breathing become more erratic. When she would open her eyes and talk, she would have the most peaceful look on her face.

On Wednesday of that week she began to mumble. "It's amazing," she said. "I'm like an eagle."

At that point, Betsy, our daughter, and I began to talk about the fact that Jeanette would see her parents, Mamaw and Papaw, as well as Daddy Jim, my father, when she crossed over into heaven.

Jeanette was still smiling when she said, "I need to see that lady."

We replied, "Soon you will see Mimi." my nearly 101-year-old mother who was dying at that time in a Nashville hospital. We believed she was the lady Jeanette said she needed to see.

"Oh, my! Oh, my!" Jeanette excitedly uttered.

While holding her hand, Betsy asked Jeanette, "Who is holding your hand?"

Fully expecting her to reply "Betsy," Jeanette surprised us when she said, "Jesus." And then Jeanette said, "That's Mama!"

"Does she look pretty?" Betsy asked.

"Yes," Jeanette said. "Are they close?"

"Yes, very close," Betsy responded. "Is your mama happy to see you?"

"Yes!" Jeanette replied.

At this point Jeanette rested a little bit and then rallied and said, "I see palm trees," and repeated that again.

Betsy asked her if she saw any iris flowers, the Tennessee state flower. Jeanette offered no response to that question. However, she went on to further describe what she was seeing: "Oh, my! Oh, my! They are all in line!"

"Everyone who loves you?" Betsy asked.

"Yes!" Jeanette replied.

A few minutes late she said, "My goodness! Those are other languages!"

"Can you understand them?" Betsy inquired.

"Yes," Jeanette smiled and said.

Jeanette said, "*Oh, my!*" three more times—for a total of seven times—in our conversation. This was an expression she normally used when something really caught her attention.

On Thursday, Jeanette slept more. She again stated she saw her mother and friends. Our hospice nurse told us, "Listen to her. She's sharing her journey with you."

I asked the nurse if this was unusual. She said it was not. She had seen it often as people neared death. That was why she advised us to pay attention, as Jeanette was acting as a guide in sharing her observations with us.

Later that day, I was standing at the foot of her bed and Jeanette looked at me, gave me the sweetest smile, slightly raised her hand, and waved at me.

The next day, Friday, Jeanette kept pointing to her left. Whatever she was seeing was happening on the left side of the room. She was trying hard to point it out to us. Her last words were: "It's soooo nice."

Her physical body shut down on Monday morning around 4:00 AM. However, I think her precious spirit went to heaven that Friday night.

While these experiences do not happen for everyone, they are not uncommon. My pastor friend Ray told me of attending to his wife in the last days of her battle with dementia. A woman of great faith, his wife had endured life-threatening experiences in her earlier years, including having a bayonet pointed at her. She believed her guardian angel had seen her safely through each incident. In the latter days of her life she was tormented with great fear, insecurity, and nightmares. She awoke one morning with a smile on her face. Ray asked her if she had not had any nightmares that night. To this she confidently replied, "My angel slept with me." The nightmares never returned.

Do not take these experiences lightly. Note them. Do not miss sharing the journey with the one you love as they slip from this world through the thin line that separates us from time and finiteness into infinity and the other side where the loving Father awaits His children's arrival home.

EXPERIENCING THE DEATH
OF YOUR LOVED ONE

Hospice will be a great help in the final hours and at the passing of your loved one. They will provide resources to help explain what is happening with your loved one as the end is near. Hospice will answer your questions and address your concerns with kind and empathetic professionalism. They will also provide a quiet and peaceful sanctuary for you and your loved ones.

Relatives play a role in helping their loved one to die with dignity. Having a prepared DNR (Do Not Resuscitate) document available, if that is your family's decision, is one of the ways you can honor the patient's previous decision on this important matter.

Deb's Experience:

I spent the last three days with my dad before he passed. During that time, I wanted to call a sibling of my father with whom he had not spoken in a long time. I asked her to come and make things right with him before he passed. When she came, I explained to her that hospice had told me Dad could still hear our voices. I encouraged her to go to his bed and speak to him. I watched and listened as she told him she was sorry, asked him to forgive her, and told him she loved him. This was a powerful healing experience for our family.

I also took advantage of those last precious days together with my dad by sharing everything my heart wanted to say to him. I told him over and over again how much I loved him. I also sang to him. I laid on the bed beside him so he would not feel alone.

When hospice shared the end was near, we called family to come, we stood in a circle around his bed and sang "Amazing Grace" and prayed together as he slipped from this life to the next.

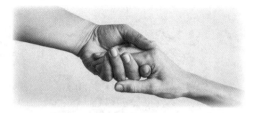

Scripture: "The time has come for my departure. I have fought the good fight. I have finished the race. I have kept the faith" (2 Timothy 4:6–7).

Prayer: *Lord of life and eternity, I release my precious one to leave the harbor of this life and set sail for a new land: the place You called "my Father's house." Home at last! Thank You, my resurrecting King!*

QUESTION #17:

WHAT THINGS MUST I DO AFTER MY LOVED ONE HAS PASSED?

THERE ARE SEVERAL important tasks to which to attend in the days and weeks following the death of your loved one:

- If your loved one was an organ donor, arrangements for this should be made immediately after death.

- If there is no organ donation or need for an autopsy, a funeral home will need to come and transport the body.

- Notify other family members and close friends.

- Contact the funeral home to make the necessary arrangements.

- Obtain multiple copies of the death certificate.

- Contact the life insurance company to make an appointment with insurance agent.

- Contact the Social Security office.

- Meet with your family attorney to take an inventory of loved one's assets and begin the process of settling the will.

- Gather financial information regarding outstanding debts and important bills that need to be settled.

- If your loved one had a financial adviser, set up a meeting to handle other financial assets.

- If you have not already done so, take your loved one's name off all financial accounts, including checking, savings, mortgage, credit cards, and title on your car.

- Close accounts, emails, reoccurring bills, subscriptions, et cetera.

- If you rented medical equipment for your loved one, you will need to call and have these items picked up.

- If your loved one lived alone, consider having their mail forwarded. Make the necessary arrangements to deal with perishable items that need to be thrown away. Other items (e.g., check books, personal information with account numbers, jewelry, and other valuable items) will need to be removed.

- Write thank-you notes as needed. Writing notes to those who have helped your loved one and you make it through this journey can help you in your grieving and healing process.

- After your loved one has passed, allow yourself to part with special things in the timing that is right for you by giving them to people you know, or to whom your loved one would want to have them.

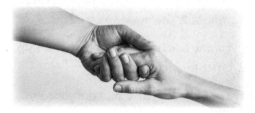

Scripture: "Now the dwelling of God is with men, and He will live with them. He will wipe every tear from their eyes. There will be no more death and mourning or crying or pain, for the old order of things has passed away" (Revelation 21:3–4).

Prayer: *Alpha and Omega, I am deeply grateful that my loved one is no longer chained to a broken mind and body. I am counting on You to see me through the valley of the shadow of death.*

QUESTION #18:

HOW DO I MOVE
FORWARD WITH MY LIFE?

G RIEVING IS A normal and healthy part of dealing with the loss of a loved one. Allow yourself time and privacy to grieve. This will be different for everyone. Seek the guidance of a trusted counselor if you need help processing your grief.

RESTORING HOPE IN MY LIFE

This slow, hard journey with your loved one battling AD will have depleted a great deal of your positive feelings. You may have a hard time being hopeful, as well. This is not healthy for you. As theologian Emil Brunner said, "What oxygen is to the lungs, such is hope to the meaning of life."

If you and your loved one have placed your faith in the God of all hope, God's Word is the message you need to hear and take to heart:

> *Praise be to the God and Father of our Lord Jesus Christ! In His great mercy He has given us new birth into a living hope through the resurrection of Jesus Christ from the dead* (1 Peter 1:3).

Bob Buford, a successful business executive and author, had one child named Ross. At the age of twenty-four, Ross drowned on the Rio Grande River. He called his son's death the equivalent of "a rogue wave washing

101

into our lifeboat." As Bob struggled to deal with Ross's death, a friend posed the question, "What do you have in your emotional toolbox that can help you navigate this time of deep grief?"

Bob acknowledged he had intelligence in his toolbox, but he could not think his way out of his son's death. He had wealth in his toolbox, but he could not buy his way out of his son's death. He had communication skills in his toolbox, but he could not talk his way out of his son's death. However, most importantly, he had faith in Jesus Christ in his toolbox, and concluded that his only option was to trust his way through his son's death.[1]

Trust your way through this stage of the journey. The death of our loved one is not a dead-end, nor a cul-de-sac, but a preview of the passage into our very real, eternal home.

EXPERIENCING HEALING IN MY LIFE

Following the experience of your loved one's passing, you may need another kind of experience: the healing of your emotional well-being, physical condition, as well as your relationship with God. There are two facets of your relationship with God that will tremendously impact your emotional and spiritual healing:

1. Anger with God

In 2019, an estimated 5.8 million Americans were living with Alzheimer's. By 2050, this number is projected to rise to nearly 14 million.[2] There are people from all walks of life who have been and are being affected by AD. From the president of the United States (Ronald Reagan) to the most humble worker, from the highly educated to the uneducated illiterate, and from the richest elite to the destitute refugee, millions of individuals will walk through this disease. We cannot control who will or will not be diagnosed with this horrible disease.

Prior to your loved one's being diagnosed with AD, they might appear healthy and enjoying life. Then one day, your loved one forgets something. This begins to happen more often. Next, you find your loved one struggling with memory issues on a regular basis. More and more symptoms arise. Later, they are diagnosed with a form of dementia or Alzheimer's.

When this happens, you will experience a shift in your emotions.

This shift from "normal" emotions to emotional upheaval can lead to your becoming angry. You may feel angry this happened to someone you love or angry at God that He would allow this to happen. Maybe you are angry that you will have to care for your loved one or angry that dream plans will not happen. You might even feel angry that others will know about this disease affecting your family. It is normal to feel upset if your loved one has been diagnosed with AD, especially if he or she lived a vital, healthy, and active life.

Anger is an emotion that should be dealt with in a healthy way so you can transition to a place where you can physically and emotionally care for your loved one.

2. Peace with God

By far the most comforting thing for me and my family, as well as for Deb and hers, was, and still is, knowing that the loss of a loved one is not the final goodbye. Years ago, Jeanette had made the most important decision a person can ever make. She chose to receive Jesus Christ as her personal Savior.

When one makes that choice, eternal life begins. Physical death becomes the transitional stage to a place the Bible calls heaven and to a complete relationship with the One who gave His life on a cross in Jerusalem over two thousand years ago to make this a reality. Jesus promised:

> *"Do not let your hearts be troubled. Trust in God; trust also in me. In my Father's house are many rooms; if it were not so I would have told you. I am going there to prepare a place for you. I will come back and take you to be with me that you also may be where I am...I am the Way, and the Truth, and the Life"* (John 14:1–6).

Sin separates us from God. If that sin is left unforgiven by God, it eternally separates us from God. God's Son, Jesus, did something for us we cannot do for ourselves. He took our place and paid the price for our sin by dying on a cross. He did this so we can be forgiven and live forever with Him.

This is a gift we can accept if we acknowledge our sin and our desperate need for Him. We must trust Him. Receive the greatest gift of peace with God who offers you His forgiveness and love.

Perhaps you need to release anger tied to this disease or take off other heavy burdens of your heart. You should not try to handle life alone. You do not need to be weighed down by feelings of inadequacy or guilt. Acknowledge your need of a Savior. Believe Jesus died for the sins of the world and accept His accomplished work on the Cross as God's gift of love to you.

My Jeanette accepted Jesus as a young girl. Deb's dad was also a believer in Christ. You, too, can know the relationship that is above all other relationships. A true relationship with our living Lord is most rewarding. He will be with you, help lighten your load, and see you through the days ahead. Remember, *"The peace of God, which transcends all understanding, will guard you hearts and minds in Christ Jesus"* (Philippians 4:7). This wonderful peace will be your daily companion as you walk this difficult road with your loved one. His Presence will be with you now and forever!

LIVING THE NEXT CHAPTER OF YOUR LIFE

Upon our return from the memorial service and burial of Jeanette in Nashville, my daughter and son-in-law dropped me off in the late evening at my home in Orlando. As we were traveling home, I could not believe all that had transpired. The last month seemed like a blur.

My mother passed away four days before Jeanette had gone to heaven. I had dashed to Nashville to say good-bye to Mom and tell her how much I loved her. I was unable to stay long as I had to hurry back to Orlando to be with Jeanette in her last days. I left Jeanette again to return to Nashville to preach at my mother's home-going celebration. I then quickly returned to Orlando to be with Jeanette. After her passing, we had a reception at the church for the hundreds who came to pay their respects to Jeanette and grieve with us. I preached at my beloved Jeanette's memorial service in Orlando,[3] returned to Nashville for a memorial service for Jeanette with friends and loved ones who live there, and then buried Jeanette's "tired tent" into the cold, hard ground beside my mom and dad at our family plot at the Spring Hill Cemetery.

Utterly exhausted when my daughter and son-in-law dropped me off at home, I entered the dark, quiet house to realize the absence of the face and voice I had cherished for sixty-two years. The silence was deafening. The house without the one who had made it *our home* felt indescribably void of the love that had filled its rooms.

In that moment home alone became my new normal. So many "no mores" raced through my head:

- No more meds to purchase and pills to sort

- No more shuffling feet and soiled garments

- No more reading the Bible, praying, and kissing good morning and good night

- No more hearing my beloved's saying "I love you"

- No more touch of her hands on my body

- No more holding hands while watching golf tournaments

- No more pushing a wheelchair to church or to EPCOT's Candlelight Processional

- No more feeding her one bite at a time at dinner

- No more seeing her searching eyes trying to comprehend

- No more of her not recognizing this man she knew but did not know

In addition to these "no mores," came a flood of over a half-century of memories of our shared lives. I cried as my new normal began.

As you begin your new normal after the passing of your loved one, you may experience some of the following:

- Your grief will continue. It will pop up unexpectedly: looking at a picture, handling a piece of clothing, sitting in church, hearing a song you both loved.

- You initially will receive lots of expressions of love, attention, and prayers. The notes, cards, emails, and texts may be sent to you for months.

- Allow yourself time to go out and be with family and friends without feeling guilty. However, expect to feel like a "fifth wheel" if you lost your spouse when you go out with friends who still have their spouses.

- You will find it uncomfortable to go to a restaurant, ask for a "table for one," and eat alone if you lost your spouse.

- You will need to go through closets and dispense of clothing, personal affects, and other items no longer needed. Do this at your own pace.

- You will want to hold on to legacy pieces—jewelry, Bible, letters, pictures, furniture, art, et cetera—to pass onto family and friends.

- You may find yourself doing unusual things as you seek to hold onto memories of your loved one. For example, I kept several of Jeanette's favorite dresses to remind me of her. I would occasionally smell them in attempt to sense a feeling of her presence.

- You may dream of your loved one. I have had dreams in which I have seen Jeanette.

- You need to get back to your living your life—your work, church, hobbies, friends—soon after the passing of your loved one.

- You must be determined to go on living and making a positive contribution in your family, church, business, and community.

- You should not keep from talking about your loved one. While it may evoke tears, it may also bring laughter. Share the things they said or did that left a positive impact on your life. Henry Scott-Holland[4] wrote these words in a poem:

> *Laugh as we always laughed at the little jokes we enjoyed together. Play, smile, think of me...Let my name be ever the household word that it always was.*

- You will find prayer can become a stabilizing, comforting, and encouraging factor in your life.

- You can find great comfort in reading the Bible and God's promises concerning heaven, reunion, and the fact your loved one is no longer suffering. Two examples of such Scripture are Revelation 21:3–5 and John 14:1–2.

- You can become an invaluable asset to others who are dealing with this disease and need a friend, listener, counselor, or prayer partner. You have walked this road and can speak from experience, not theory.

- You may find it takes a year or longer to settle legal and business affairs.

- You will have many other things about which you will have to make decisions as you move on with life. Life choices about keeping a home, downsizing, or moving elsewhere are important. Do not rush into these matters. Talk with wise counselors, family, or friends. Pray for guidance.

When my father died, my mother began to think about selling their house in Nashville and moving to Florida or a senior living community. My brother and I urged her to wait a year. She did and ended up staying in her home for another twenty years.

- You will find companionship important, especially if you have lost your spouse. The presence and voice of someone you respect and appreciate can soothe the rough edges of that part of your life that is now absent.

- You may find "first" birthdays, wedding anniversaries, holidays, family events, or vacations to be emotional. However, these occasions give you the opportunity to recall the joy of these special days in years gone by.

- You will find the possibility of remarriage to be something worthy of consideration if you have lost a spouse. It has been found that those who were happily married have the most difficult time in adjusting after the death of their spouse. They are most likely to be open to another marital relationship.

Both Jeanette and I were among those individuals who loved being in a marriage relationship. As many married couples might do, we discussed the proposition of remarrying from time to time, usually in a lighthearted way. I would say, "If you can find a godly man who can afford you, marry him if I pass first." She would say, "If I go first and you can find a godly woman who can put up with you, marry her."

I faced this proposition after Jeanette's death. I have since remarried. As I approached the decision to remarry, I remembered Jeanette's sharing with me a conversation she had with her father, a godly man who had lost his wife to cancer and remained single for twelve years until his death. In that conversation with Jeanette, her dad was looking back over his life and said with regret, "The biggest mistake I made was not remarrying. It's not meant for 'man to be alone.'" [5] His words proved to be helpful and wise counsel for me.

Deb's Experience:

My mom had not planned or thought of remarriage after Dad passed away. However, nine years after he passed, God brought a wonderful, godly man (whose wife had passed of cancer) into her life. They married and are enjoying life together while still cherishing the memory of their loved ones.

As a caregiver without a loved one for whom to care, life as you have known it has changed again. As you begin putting the pieces of your life back together—renewing relationships with others and with God; taking better care of yourself physically, emotionally, and spiritually; embracing each new day for the hopeful possibilities and opportunities it brings—consider these familiar words of King Solomon as written in the book of Ecclesiastes:

> *There is a time for everything,*
>   *and a season for every activity under heaven:*
>   *A time to be born and a time to die,*
>   *A time to plant and a time to uproot...*
>   *A time to tear down and a time to build,*
>   *A time to weep and a time to laugh,*
>   *A time to mourn and a time to dance...*
>   *A time to keep and a time to throw away,*
>   *A time to tear and a time to mend,*
>   *A time to be silent and a time to speak...*
> *[God] has made everything beautiful in its time.*
> *He has also set eternity in the human heart.*
>   —FROM ECCLESIASTES 3:1–11

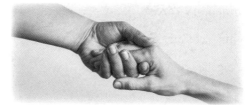

Scripture: "I will turn their mourning into gladness; I will give them comfort and joy instead of sorrow" (Jeremiah 3:13).

Prayer: *Eternal Creator—the same yesterday, today, and tomorrow—grant me the grace to cherish the good memories, move past what I can never change, and believe You are doing a new work in my life. The best is yet!*

RESOURCES

Websites

- Alzheimer's Association: Education and Referral Center, as well as financial and legal planning: www.alz.org

- Community Resource Finder: www.communityresource finder.org

- Elder Care, Support and Help: www.eldercare.acl.gov/Public/Index.aspx

- Kirby Pines LifeCare Community; Memphis, Tennessee: www.kirbypines.com

- National Hospice and Palliative Care Organization: www.nhpco.org

- National Respite Locator Service: www.archrespite.org/respitelocator

- Paying for Care: Financial Advice: www.payingforsenior care.com/memory-care

- Still Serving Veterans: Financial Advice: www.SSV.org

- Visiting Angels: www.Visitingangels.com

Books

- *The 36-Hour Day*: A Family Guide for Caring for People Who Have Alzheimer Disease, Other Dementias, and Memory Loss; Nancy L. Mace, MA, & Peter V. Rabins, MD, MPH; Johns Hopkins University Press, 2017.

- *Till Death Do Us Part*; Robertson McQuilkin; FamilyLife, 2000.

Songs

- "Ellsworth," Rascal Flatts

- "I'm Not Gonna Miss You," Glen Campbell
- "Raymond," Brett Eldredge
- "While He Still Knows Who I Am," Kenny Chesney

Videos

- *Singer Glen Campbell on his recent Alzheimer's diagnosis* (www.youtube.com)
- *The Alzheimer's Project* (HBO)

Movies

- Away from Her (Liongate Films: 2007)
- Head Full of Honey (Warner Brothers: 2019)
- Poetry (Next Entertainment World: 2011)
- Still Alice (Sony Pictures Classics, 2014)
- The Notebook (New Line Cinema: 2004)

Dementia Virtual Experience

- This company provides a virtual experience for those who want to know how AD impacts one's senses and thinking. The Alzheimer's Experience is called Second Wind Dreams (Virtual Dementia Tour); Roswell, GA; secondwind.org.

DEDICATION BY JIM HENRY

To the love of my life, Jeanette Sturgeon Henry, whose love for Jesus, the Bible, and me never wavered under the withering ravages of Alzheimer's. Her courage in the face of an illness that robbed her of so much but could not destroy her determined effort to stare down this relentless enemy was inspiring. Her faith was undaunted as it waded through questions, fears, a changing world, tears, and uncertainty, but stayed anchored to the Rock of Ages. She, who not by her choice, but in the providence of God, gave me the privilege of being her primary caregiver, which if I had known sixty years ago was to be my lot, I would have volunteered for that privilege a thousand times over.

And to God's angel caregivers—Betsy Henry de Armas, Arlicia Coleman, Kathy Siegel Henry, Laura Daniele, Marion Daniele, Mary Williams Condon, Dawn Harris, and Suzanne Feil—whose compassionate care demonstrated the heart of God, gave me a break from the demands of the "36-hour day,"[1] and refreshed me during the constantly evolving changes that were happening in our lives, I thank you with all my heart.

DEDICATION BY DEB TERRY

To MY DAD, Ray J. Denney, who helped shape my life through his kind, loving, and tender ways. Through his faith, discipline, and strong work ethic, he fought to the end, bringing great encouragement and strength to me as one of his caregivers during the darkest days of his life. He taught me well! My life will forever be changed because I had the honor to help care for you, my dad, whom I love so deeply.

To the many family members, friends, and caregivers who loved my dad and were champions in his care, I thank you. To my husband, Scott, for your constant unconditional love and support; my mom, June, my hero from whom I learned so much about life, death, faith and marriage by watching her unconditional love and care for Dad; and to my brother, Steve, and his wife, Vickie: Dad would have been so proud of you and how we all worked together. To the grandchildren and great-grandchildren whom loved Dad well; to Berry and Betty Terry, my in-laws, for their help and support; to great friends including Jack and Patsy Bolton; to Dr. Alfred Ratcliffe, Jr., a family physician and friend; to Dr. J. Russell Robinson, Dad's primary and hospice physician; and to Annette Marlar, the Director of Medical Service, and her team of caregivers at Job's Way, I am indebted to each one of you. I did not want to waste the pain. Instead, it is my desire to use it to bring honor and glory to my heavenly Father, as well as offer help and hope to others traveling this journey. I am blessed that God allowed me to be the daughter of Ray J. Denney and call him *Dad*!

ACKNOWLEDGMENTS

From Jim Henry

To Deb Terry, former member of our leadership team at First Baptist Church, Orlando, who sent me an email after Jeanette's death and asked if I had considered writing something to assist caregivers of Alzheimer's patients. When I asked why, she told me two things. First, she had been praying for years about helping people going through this journey. As her family had walked that long road, she did not want to waste the experience, rather she wanted to do something positive in honor of her beloved father. Second, while she was praying about it, the Holy Spirit spoke to her and nudged her to get in touch with me. I did not dare ignore that prompting! Thank You, Holy Spirit. Thank you, Deb, for your wonderful contributions and passion to make this book a reality.

To Marilyn Jeffcoat whose skills, enthusiasm, and tireless work to pull all of our material into a concise and focused product, and who, by prayer and sensitivity to the Spirit of God, shaped our words into arrows that will pierce the clouds of fear, doubt, and uncertainty that surround us when we walk this path with our loved ones. We know these words you helped to craft will shatter that darkness with hope, help, and healing. Thanks, Marilyn, our benevolent taskmaster.

To Kris Den Besten, who jumped in immediately with a "let's make it happen" when he heard about our project. The business expertise he brought to the table, the wisdom he imparted, and the support he afforded us were indispensable in propelling our venture to this threshold. Thank you, Kris.

To our go-to cover designer, artist, and friend, Dee DeLoy, who poured not only his artistic skill into our project but his heart for serving the Lord and others. Dee beautifully conveyed with his photography and artwork what we are trying to say with our words.

To all of you who through the years who held up our spirits and our arms with your prayers, cards, emails, texts, and willingness to share our burdens, only heaven knows the times that those caring actions were like a cold drink in the dry, dusty, and dirty desert we were crossing. Great is our gratitude. Great will be your reward. Thank you with all my heart.

From Deb Terry

To "Bro Jim" Henry, a wonderful ministry leader and example of humility. I will forever be grateful God allowed me the opportunity to serve the Lord Jesus with you at First Baptist Church of Orlando. It was a joy to be under your tutelage. I am so thankful God connected our lives, and the power of the Holy Spirit led us to partner together in ministry and co-author this book. I am thankful for this opportunity to share our experiences and how our faith carried us through as caregivers to our loved ones with Alzheimer's with you for Jeanette and me for Ray. Thank you for reading my email, praying, and saying *yes* to this book! I will forever be grateful. To God be the glory!

To Marilyn Jeffcoat, a gifted, creative woman who loves Jesus and His Word, and a precious friend always finding a way to encourage me to be my best while fulfilling God's purpose in my life. You are masterful with words and finding a way for them to capture a reader's heart. Thank you for being a great teacher as I was writing my first book.

To Kris Den Besten, who is a champion for sharing God's love with purpose and passion. Your heart and generosity is huge and inspires me. Thanks for showing up, listening, and providing great insight and assistance. You are a "make-it-happen," godly man.

To Annette Marlar, whose heart, compassion and professionalism as a health care leader profoundly impacted my life and this book. You and your team found ways to love and care for my dad, Ray, like no other team was able to do. You planted the seed in my heart to write this book. Thank you and Kirby Pines Life Care Community for helping me not waste the pain of this experience.

For information on ordering this book or
contacting the authors, visit their websites:

Jim Henry: www.jimhenry.today

Deb Terry: www.debdterry.com

ABOUT THE AUTHORS

Dr. James B. (Jim) Henry is one of the most respected Christian leaders of our day. The author of eight books, Dr. Henry is a popular speaker and conference leader. Completing two terms as the president of the Southern Baptist Convention, this denominational leader serves on numerous boards and commissions throughout the United States. A graduate of Georgetown College and New Orleans Baptist 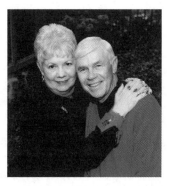 Theological Seminary, he served as the senior pastor of the mega church First Baptist Church in Orlando for twenty-nine years. Residing in Orlando, Dr. Henry enjoys golfing, reading, traveling, and spending time with his family.

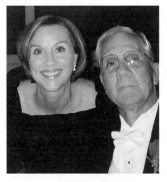 **Deborah "Deb" Denney Terry** was born in Albertville, Alabama, where she lived for most of her life. Deb is fulfilling God's calling on her life to serve Him in vocational ministry: first, through music ministry as a singer-songwriter and recording artist; second, through serving in various ministry positions in churches in Alabama and Florida, which she has done for over twenty years. Formerly the Director of Children's Ministry at Meadowbrook Baptist Church in Alabama and then at First Baptist Church in Orlando, Deb and her husband, Scott, currently reside in Central Florida, where Deb serves on the staff of Winter Garden's First Baptist Church as Director of their second campus and Women's Ministry. She and Scott have two children who are married. They have five amazing grandchildren. Deb enjoys her family, music, reading, and travel.

NOTES

Preface

1. Vince Gil, *When I Call Your Name*, MCA Records, 1989.

Question #1:
What Are the First Things I Need to Know?

1. Medical review by Neil Lava, MD, "Ten Early Signs of Alzheimer's," *Web*MD Medical Reference, 5 May 2019.

2. Your local Alzheimer's Association or Alzheimer's Disease Center can help in finding a specialist.

3. "Types of Dementia," Dementia/Understand Together, understandtogether website, 3 January 2020.

4. Jeff Howard, "Dementia vs. Alzheimer's Disease: Biggest Differences to Remember, activebeat.com website, 4 January 2020.

5. "The Three Most Common Types of Dementia and Their Differences," AssistedLivingToday.com, updated 30 October 2019.

Question #2:
What Are the First Steps I Need to Take?

1. Medical review by Timothy J. Legg, Ph.D., CRNP, "Life Expectancy and Long-Term Outlook for Alzheimer's Disease, *Healthline* website, 13 October 2016.

Question #3:
How Do I Share the Diagnosis?

1. No author cited, "Sharing the Diagnosis," Alzheimer's Association website: alz.org, 4 January 2020.

Question #5:
Who Can Help Me Get Through This?

1. Jennifer Wegerer, "The Five Best Emotional Support Groups for Alzheimer's Caregivers," Alzheimer's.net, 13 March 2019.

Question #6:
What Roles Must I Assume to Protect My Loved One?

1. Marlis Powers, "Dementia Patients Need an Advocate," *AgingCare* website, 6 January 2020.

2. Ibid.

Question #7:
What Financial and Legal Preparation Do I Need to Make?

1. Marlo Sollitto, "Family Caregivers Bear the Burden of High Elder Care Costs," *AgingCare* website, updated 17 June 2019.

2. "The Financial Burden of Alzheimer's for Caregivers," *Alzheimers.net* website, 1 December 2019.

3. "The Financial Burden of Alzheimer's for Caregivers," *Alzheimers.net* website, 1 December 2019.

4. "Alzheimer's Disease Facts and Figures," Alzheimer's Association website: alz.org, 6 January 2020.

5. "The Financial Burden of Alzheimer's for Caregivers," *Alzheimers.net* website, 1 December 2019.

6. "New York Cost of Care 2018 Survey," AARP website, 1 December 2019.

7. Ibid.

8. Ibid.

Question #8:
What Can I Do to Prolong the Good Years?

1. "Jeanette Henry - Celebration of Life" on YouTube, February 2019.

2. Vic Jacobson in a note to his supporters, n.d.

Question #9:
How Do I Tackle the Daily Care of My Loved One?

1. For example, Silverts: www.silverts.com (adaptive clothing).

2. Jonathan Graff-Radford, "Sundowning: Late-Day Confusion," *Mayo Clinic* website, 8 January 2020.

Question #10:
How Do I Handle Negative Personality Changes?

1. No author cited, "How to Handle Personality Changes and Aggression," *Dementia.org* website, 8 January 2020.

2. No author cited, "Depression," Alzheimer's Association website: alz.org, 8 January 2020.

3. Jeanne Murray Walter, "Mother in Late Bloom," *Christianity Today*, July/August 2014.

4. Fr. *Parade Magazine*, 14 July 2009.

QUESTION #11:
HOW MIGHT I IMPROVE MY LOVED ONE'S QUALITY OF LIFE?

1. Louise Penny, "The Last Promise," *AARP Magazine/Real Possibilities*, p. 72; n.d.

QUESTION #12:
HOW DO I TAKE CARE OF MYSELF?

1. No author cited, "10 Symptoms of Caregiver Stress," Alzheimer's Association website: alz.org, 9 January 2020.
2. 1999 study by Stanford University cited by Toula Wooten, "When the Caregiver Is Sicker Than the Loved One," *nextavenue.org*website, 22 June 2017.

QUESTION #18:
HOW DO I MOVE FORWARD WITH MY LIFE?

1. Jay Wolf, from his pastor's column in First Baptist Church bulletin, Montgomery, Alabama, 18 January 2015.
2. Alzheimer's Disease Facts and Figures," Alzheimer's Association website: alz.org, 6 January 2020.
3. Jeanette Henry - Celebration of Life" on YouTube, February 2019.
4. Henry Scott-Holland, fr. a sermon entitled "Death of the King of Terrors," London, England, 1910.
5. Reference to Genesis 2:18.

DEDICATION BY JIM HENRY

1. Reference to the book, *The 36-Hour Day* by Nancy L. Mace and Peter V. Rabins (Johns Hopkins University Press).

INDEX

IF YOU'RE A FAN OF THIS BOOK, PLEASE TELL OTHERS...

➢ Post a 5-star review on Amazon.

➢ Write about the book on your Facebook, Twitter, Instagram, LinkedIn, or any social media platforms you regularly use.

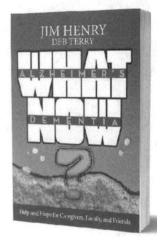

➢ If you blog, consider referencing the book or publishing an excerpt from the book with a link back to our websites. You have permission to do this as long as you provide proper credit and backlinks.

➢ Recommend the book to friends, family, and AD caregivers—word-of-mouth is still the most effective form of advertising.

➢ Purchase additional copies to give away to others or for use by your church or other groups.

➢ Learn more about the authors or contact them at...

Jim Henry: www.jimhenry.today
Deb Terry: www.debdterry.com

ENJOY THESE OTHER BOOKS BY JIM HENRY

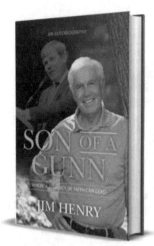

Son of a Gunn – Where a Journey of Faith Can Lead (An Autobiography)

You will laugh, you will cry, you will wonder at the greatness of the God who can take a life of a willing believer and place him at the crossroads of major events in human affairs. Jim Henry's life story is filled with insights and truths that if embraced will help your own life journey be lived with greater significance, purpose, and joy.

Keeping Life in Perspective – Sharpening Your Sense of What's Important

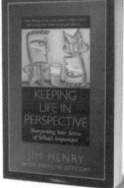

This book describes how to live life to the fullest and appreciate every minute now, instead of waiting impatiently for the perfect job, the dream house, or the million-dollar inheritance that never comes. Impatience, greed, and other evils threaten our happiness by constantly making us wish for more.

You can order these books from **www.jimhenry.today**, or wherever you purchase your favorite books.

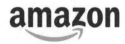
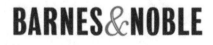